How To Achieve A 10/10 Relationship

How To Achieve A 10/10 Relationship

Once you master the five pillars of a successful relationship, you'll find your "happily ever after" with your partner.

Jake Maddock

How To Achieve A 10/10 Relationship

Once you master the five pillars of a successful relationship, you'll find your "happily ever after" with your partner.

2024 Edition

ISBN 978-1-5445-4130-3 *Hardcover*
978-1-5445-4131-0 *Paperback*
978-1-5445-4132-7 *Ebook*

Contents

PART VI: EXPANDING ON THE FIVE PILLARS

Introduction

**Great job getting the updated 2024 version, this will
help dramatically in your life.
Remember two main goals here, to help you become a
10/10 person and to help you achieve a 10/10
relationship!**

Want to have a 10/10 relationship? Want to find your ideal partner? Want to have the perfect relationship?

If you answered "yes" to any of those questions, then you are reading the right book.

For most of us, no amount of physical pain even comes close to the emotional pain of a really bad relationship. I know this from personal experience. That's why I've dedicated my life to preventing others from going through the same pain I did. Now, I am a world-class relationship coach, and I've helped people all over the world achieve the relationships they want and deserve. The typical type of client I coach is a 46-year-old female, who is divorced with kids. The majority of people I coach are single mums; they are great people but seem to have a lot of trouble with femininity, tend to overthink a lot, and have fears. I love helping and watching these people achieve a 10/10 relationship.

Because I've coached so many people from all different backgrounds, cultures, and religions, I've developed tried-and-true methods that transcend differences and speak to the very thing which makes us all human. After years of coaching, I have discovered five pillars to achieving a 10/10 relationship, which I'll outline for you in this book.

If you master these five pillars, then you will be a master at relationships. Throughout this book, you will see how I have mastered them and how my clients have, too. I will lay out very clearly everything you need to do to find your ideal partner and get the relationship to a 10/10 and keep it there forever. I hope you will apply this knowledge to your own life and become a master of relationships just like me.

WARNING

Some of the things I say in this book may offend you, or you may not agree with them. I do not apologise, and I am not sorry. Guess what. Life isn't fucking fair! Love isn't fucking fair, and the reason your past relationships have failed is because of you. Every single person I work with achieves a 10/10 relationship because I push them, and I tell them what they need to hear. I'm not going to give you a hug when you're crying and tell you you're doing a good job.

I am a no-nonsense type of coach. I push people, and sometimes I am mean. But the results speak for themselves. So if you are a delicate little flower who needs kisses and hugs constantly and likes to hold hands with people and cry, maybe this book isn't for you. So put the fucking book down and go and watch a romantic comedy while eating ice cream and complaining about how fat you are.

If you are strong enough, have an open mind, and are willing to learn and not play the victim role, then keep reading. I don't care at all if you enjoy this book; however, I do hope you learn something about relationships and about life that will improve your current situation and give you the chance to help others.

PART I

Masculine and Feminine Energy

Masculine and Feminine Energy

A masculine man and a feminine woman are truly super heroes. Especially when they are in a relationship together. Here is a little secret that most people don't know, masculine and feminine energy is kind of like a see-saw or a set of scales, as one side goes up the other goes down, which means when a woman is truly in her feminine energy then it will naturally push the man into his masculine energy. This is one of things I love about this, once I show a woman how to embrace her femininity then the man in her life feels so empowered and supported that he becomes so much happier and the relationship improves dramatically.

When a man is in his masculine energy a woman will feel safe around him, when a woman is in her feminine energy a man will feel safe around her. This sense of safety really gives a chance for love to blossom. It is very difficult for love to blossom when a man isn't masculine or a woman isn't feminine. I'm sure you have experienced this first hand just like I did. I was in terrible relationships in the past before I met my beautiful wife, where we would constantly bash heads, always fighting, like a massive power struggle. I wasn't embracing masculine energy properly and she wasn't embracing femininity properly, this was over a decade ago and gave me enough pain to begin learning, now here we are. Once someone truly learns how to embody masculine or feminine energy then nothing and no one can take them out of it, they always stay in that energy forever, it is a beautiful thing. Important to remember that these skills aren't just for your romantic partner they are from everything and everyone, from your kids to the waitress, use it everywhere and your life will be richer than you could imagine.

Unfortunately we are all humans and are at the mercy to a certain degree to our environments, having a bulletproof mindset is very important for success but if you're not very good at designing good environments for yourself then success will evade you. Truly stepping into your masculine or feminine energy respectfully is impossible if your environment is no good, because you must feel safe to be in your energy then you must ensure your environment is one that sets you up for success. In other words if you're in an absolutely terrible relationship with the wrong person then it will seem almost impossible to be in your energy properly. I see this everyday, I coach many couples from all around the world and I always see one of two things, either a couple who can get to a 10/10 or a couple who can't, it is surprisingly easy to tell. The couple which can get to a 10/10 are willing to do whatever it takes to get the results they want and have an open mind and it is clear that they are with their ideal partner, and ideal partner being someone who you share good compatibility, chemistry and x-factor with. The couple which is doomed to fail are often extremely stubborn and it is clear they are definitely not with their ideal partner.

If you're in a relationship with someone who is clearly not your ideal partner then you will never truly be able to embrace your masculine or feminine energy properly. Unfortunately I can't make this decision for you, I need you to look at your partner and truly ask yourself some hard questions, is this really my ideal partner? Can I truly get a 10/10 relationship with this person? If the answer is no then it's time to go. Remember you're better off being single than with the wrong person.

Work environments can also affect masculine and feminine energy, I hear women say everyday to me that they work in a male dominated workplace, I understand this can definitely feel like it makes it a lot harder, maybe feels like you need to become one of the boys. This is not the case, becoming one of the boys won't make your career progress faster, it will just leave you being disliked. Here is a very very important point to remember, if you aren't like then you aren't heard!

In other words if you want to be heard, you want to be listened to, you want influence then you must be likable to a certain degree. A woman in her masculine energy is not heard and is disliked, she is doing herself a massive disservice. I coach about 70% single mums and a common thing I hear every day is, oh, I'm a single mum so I've had to do both roles, mum and dad. Just out of curiosity how is that working out? I bet it's not very good, a mum stepping into her masculine energy in an attempt to be a more effective parent is silly, being overly aggressive will only yield short term results but long term failure. Being a feminine mum will yield much better results, your kids will like you more so they will listen and they will want to be part of your life for many decades.

As you can see masculine and feminine energy has a lot to do with mindset and emotion. If you have a bad mindset, if you let fear consume your thoughts, if you lack confidence and courage then stepping into the right energy will almost seem impossible. As many of you know I help people achieve 10/10 relationships, but in reality the main thing I do is help people become a 10/10 within who they are. Once I help people become a 10/10 within themselves than they are 90% of the way to success. So what does this include? To put it simply if you have low self esteem and no confidence then stepping into your masculine or feminine energy will seem impossible. It takes courage to proudly step into your energy, so it is essential, but how do we build that up?

First step is self-talk, our words have so much power and they are so underestimated. Some common negative self talk people say is -

- I'm no good at being feminine

- Masculine and Feminine energy is stupid, I don't need that

- My situation is hopeless, nothing can help me now

- I suffer with anxiety

- I've always been bad at this

These kind of sentences concrete failure as your only option in life. Never talk ill of yourself. Some people argue saying well if I just said positive affirmations all the time wouldn't that be lying? Well who's to say that those negative sentences are the true? It's merely your own perception, those negative things are your truth because you have said them ten thousands times. Now it's time to say some positive sentences ten thousand times, notice how much your life will change when you are in control and intentionally chose the words you say. Remember your words become your thoughts which become your reality. Many people think it starts with your thoughts but really how many humans put that much thought into our words? Not many, most people just talk talk talk without thinking much about it, nevertheless if it's positive or negative. The reality is the more ill things about yourself you say, the more negative sentence you spew out the harder it will be to be successful in whatever you are trying to do, weather it's sport, relationships or a business, a positive attitude will make achieve your goals far easier and quicker.

As you remember the opposite to masculine and feminine energy is fear. Fear is the most expensive emotion, it will take more from than any other emotion. A big part of what I teach in my program is emotional maturity, which means choosing the emotion you want to feel. Sounds crazy hey! How could it be so simple? Well it is! So I want you to think to yourself, what emotion do I want to feel tomorrow?

When I ask myself this question, this is the answer I get - Tomorrow I want to feel - grateful, enthusiastic, happy, joyful, strong, masculine, lucky, loved, appreciated, respected, generous, powerful, handsome, wise, intelligent, successful. They are some of the things which come to mind. Take a notepad and pen and write down how you want to feel tomorrow. Intentionally choosing your emotions is one of smartest things you can do! If you become a master of your emotions then your life will be absolutely amazing and you will be able to stay in your masculine or feminine energy better because remember how fear is the opposite of masculine and feminine energy? If you intentionally choose your emotion then you won't choose fear will you! As you can see, mindset plays into these energies so strongly, with a strong mindset you can achieve anything.

I truly believe if everyone in the world read this book then the world would be a better place, with masculine and feminine energy there are 4 behavioral traits I want you to try to envelop into your day to day lives. If you are a man, I want you to be more masculine, those masculine traits being - Leadership, Ambition, Decisiveness and Protection. If you are a woman, I want you to be more feminine, those feminine traits being - Nurturing, Supportive, Caring and Joyous. If you embody these traits well then you will feel like a superhero, your life and the peoples lives around you will improve dramatically! Let's break down what it all really means, what's the true purpose of all this?

Masculine Energy - Purpose - To provide strength and overall leadership.

Feminine Energy - Purpose - To create love and desire.

As you can see very different purposes to either energies. Men and women are very different. One of the most ridiculous questions I have ever been asked is, do you think men and women are equal? This question is so absurd! It's like asking, are bananas and oranges equal? Or are dogs and cats equal? What?! Firstly, why are they competing against each other? They are completely different things, I love bananas and I love oranges, one isn't better, however they are both very different and both have their pros and cons. Men and women are very different, both are great, both deserve the utmost respect. Trying to make men and women the same has been an unwise move of the 21st century which truly only seems to serve the government and the taxes they collect; however that is only a short term win on their side and long term we all lose. But enough about politics, I'm here to teach you how to step into your energy and why, not on the things that current cultures and societies are doing wrong which is making it harder to be in your respected energy.

As you can see it would've been very easy for me to sit here and write a hundred thousand words on all the ways the world is making it harder for the average person to step into their masculine and feminine energy, but I have spent years working on having a brilliant bulletproof mindset, so I FOCUS on what I want to achieve, not what I want to avoid. Write that sentence down for me. Because it ties very well back into emotions. If you are getting a lot of negative emotional feedback in your life it is most likely because you are focused on what you want to avoid and not what you want to achieve. If you focus on what you want to avoid you will feel fear, anxiety, stress, all the bad stuff.

If you focus on what you want to achieve you will feel enthusiasm, excitement, joy, hope, all the good stuff. Focus is extremely important and a big part in having a brilliant mindset and staying in your masculine or feminine energy.

The purpose of masculine energy is to provide strength and overall leadership. This is extremely important, if a man does this well then his wife will feel safe and loved and it will allow her to easily and comfortably step into her feminine energy and stay there. If he does not do this well then the relationship will feel like a rollercoaster, she will not feel safe, she will be full of fear, and her walls will go up causing her to jump out of her feminine energy therefore causing the attraction in the relationship to plummet. The masculine man is emotionally mature, he is in control of his emotions, he is focused on what he needs to achieve and knows how to be a fantastic leader.

The most important trait of a masculine man is his ability to lead, but what does it really mean to be a great leader? He needs to lead his family to success, lead his relationship to a 10/10, and lead his family to better tomorrow. He takes full responsibility for the things which happen around him and full responsibility for his family and relationship. He is there to serve his family, he is there to do what is best. Trying to be as humble as possible, I am a great leader, through many years of practice. The people I lead aren't there to serve me, I am there to serve them, I am responsible for their well being and their success, if they fail, then I have failed. The people I lead can not truly fail, if they fail then I take the responsibility of failure however if they will I let them have the victory themselves. Being a true leader isn't always so glamorous, I am truly honored I can be a great leader and help make people's lives better. A leader must have a solid foundation of integrity and always doing what I right isn't always the most fun, as a leader I've had to do many things I didn't really want to do, have many conversations that I didn't want to have, but because I have intentional choose my identity, I have no fear and I am masculine man, that means doing the right thing regardless of how hard it is because that is the best thing for the team, family, relationship, community and so on. If you are a man reading this then you must know, you must be a masculine man if you want to achieve a 10/10 relationship or a successful business or successful life, it is not optional. Unfortunately as sexist as it may sound, men must be the leader in the relationship, if a woman is the leader then the relationship will never be a 10/10. I really wish this wasn't the case because I hate sounding sexist, I really love women and think they are great but every single relationship I've seen where the woman is the leader was at best a 7/10 relationship. I have coached so many couples where the woman is masculine and the man is feminine, they are so unhappy, butting heads all the time, it's terrible, as soon as I teach them how to do it properly and swap them back around it gets to a 10/10 and everyone is super happy again. So if you're a woman and you feel offended right now, don't stress, keep reading, I'm here to help you achieve a 10/10 you and a 10/10 relationship, trust the process and listen to what I have to say.

To break it down simply guys, leadership is about taking full responsibility for you and all those around you at all times, never giving excuses and having solid integrity, integrity means doing what you believe is best for yourself, your family, the community and the universe. All four circles getting bigger and bigger and remember is what YOU think is best, not what I think is best for you. Men this is essential for you to do ok, if you as a man can become truly masculine then it will make the world a better place. That covers leadership, the next trait of masculinity that I want men to embrace is ambition! Having goals is super important, a lazy man is very unattractive, men you must have goals and dreams, a vision for a better tomorrow. Nothing worse than seeing a man with no drive, no goals, no ambitions, no dreams, just a real loser sitting around waiting for life to happen. As a man your goals can't be big enough, aim for the stars, be overly ambitious, go all in, 110%! That drive, that passion, that unwavering purpose is very attractive to people and the reason we have the amazing world we have today, because our forefathers were so ambitious and driven. It's not easy to build a bridge, it's not easy to build a plane or a car but our forefathers did it, they did it with passion and drive, while losers sat around and called them crazy, they worked hard, never wavering from their goals, they worked hard and tirelessly to achieve their goals regardless of what others said about them. Remember guys, the opposite to success isn't failure, the opposite to success mediocrity. You will fail many times on the path to achieving a goal, in my program where I coach people on how to achieve a 10/10 relationship, most people go on around 15 first dates, you could say there was 15 failures until meeting that ideal partner where you could succeed in creating that 10/10 relationship, but it wasn't really 15 failures was it because all the things that were learnt along the way, when I coach someone and they go on 15 first dates over 3 months that person changes a lot! They become way more confident, more interesting and a way better conversationalist! The journey to success shapes us and we become the success on the way to achieving our goals, it's truly an amazing thing to see.

It appears that the true failures in life are the people who settle for mediocrity, most people settle for a 6/10 relationship and a 6/10 career and a 6/10 life in general! It's not terrible, it's just ok. That is a failure to me! Now with ambition, the only thing that can kill ambition is fear, as we covered earlier, fear is by far the most expensive emotion, it freezes people in their tracks, it says to the loser sitting in his mum's basement, "what's the point of trying, might as well just keep playing this video game." The fears, the doubts, the insecurities, caring what others will think of you, all these things slowly corroding the ambition in your soul. A masculine man stands up, and say no! A masculine man will not be held back by fears or insecurities, he doesn't care what others think about him, he stands up and goes after his dream, his goals with full aggression and drive, he makes no plan B, he makes plan A work. He lands on the island and burns the boats behind him, he will win or die trying, that is ambition, that is drive, that is masculinity.

So we have leadership, ambition, decisiveness and protection. Decisiveness is fairly straight forward, the ability to make a decision quickly, successful people make a decision in 3 seconds, 99.99% of decisions you already have enough information to know what the right decision is, unfortunately most people lack the self confidence to make a decision quickly and feel they need to think about it for 3 days first, which is absolutely ridiculous. It takes two things to make a decision quickly, information and courage. If you have enough data on the thing and the confidence then you should be able to make a decision in 3 seconds, I even make quite hard decisions very quickly by trusting my gut, listening to your intuition and then backing yourself in your decision making is very important. Successful people make a decision quickly then take a long time to change their mind, idiots take a long time to make a decision then change their mind quickly. Remember most ideas can be good if the execution is good enough but even the best idea can fail from a lack of commitment. So there is a new test for you guys. Make every decision, regardless of how big or small in 3 seconds, you will be surprised how easy it is and how well everything turns out. Now the question is ladies, what if your man is very decisive? Well you can help him, often men are so used to being downtrodden that they think that any decision they make will turn out badly and they will be criticised for it so they rather push that responsibility onto others, know as a woman you can turn this around, if a decision needs to be made, like what to eat for dinner for example, then simply don't decide, he must decide, and keep pushing it back onto him, tell him that you want him to decide what to have and whatever he chooses you will love, keep pushing the responsibility onto him and giving him the reassurance that you will support and love him no matter what. As a woman you have the ability to push men into their masculine energy if you choose to, which you definitely should.

The last trait of masculine energy that I want men to embrace is being protective. All men should strive to be sheepdogs. Let me explain for those who don't know what that means, there are 3 types of people in the world: sheep, wolves and sheepdogs. Sheep are people who can't or choose not to defend themselves. Wolves are predators, bullies, those who prey on sheep and take advantage of the weak. Sheepdogs protect the sheep from the wolves, they fight for those who cannot fight for themselves, every man should strive to be a sheepdog, in fact I teach men and women to be sheepdogs, regardless of your gender or age I want everyone to strive to be a sheepdog, I don't thing is good to be a sheep or a wolf, the honorable thing to be in life is a sheepdog. In life realistically there won't be many opportunities where a man gets to protect his wife physically from a real physical threat, today's society is fairly safe from physical danger, however physically isn't the only way we can protect someone, you can also protect them emotionally. So for example let's say you are at a family picnic and someone makes a joke at your wife's expense, they are teasing your wife about how silly she is, fairly harmless but nevertheless a good opportunity to protect, as man that is my cue to stand up and say, no, I think my wife is very smart actually. It will shut everyone up pretty fast, some people may say this shows a lack of class or decorum in certain settings. Well I say too damn with being polite, I protect my family and stand up for others, that means more to me than being polite. As a man I want you to take every single opportunity possible to be protective, if you get the opportunity to protect then use it wisely, that is a gift from god to prove yourself, use it, tackle the opportunity aggressively and show everyone how amazing you are, never ever ever cower from opportunity to be protective, fight like you have nothing to lose, fight like you are invincible, these moments earn you deep respect from your love ones.

These are the four traits of masculinity that every man should embrace 110%. Men, if you embrace leadership, ambition, decisiveness and protection then your life will dramatically improve in every area. Embracing this with integrity is truly key to success, remember integrity is doing what you think is best, not what anyone else thinks.

The purpose of feminine energy is to create love and desire, see the main difference there? Masculine energy provides and feminine energy creates, that is an important distinction. If a woman embodies feminine energy correctly she will create deep love and strong desire around her, you see this very clearly with feminine women, they have many friends, beautiful family and are vibrant loved members of the community, everyone seems to have the desire to want to spend time with them and be in their presence. Men are deeply drawn to feminine women, even if a woman isn't particularly good looking, if she really embodies that beautiful feminine energy then men will want to be around her. Many women are very concerned with making themselves look perfect, and conventionally they may look very beautiful, they look they are straight out of a magazine but they are so masculine that men avoid them, these beautiful women think that men are intimidated because they are so beautiful, that is not the case, men don't like these women because they are masculine which is unattractive, they are definitely not intimidated, merely un-attracted. Then you will see an average looking girl but she is absolutely brimming with feminine energy and she is like a magnet, pulling everyone in, her smile lights up the room, while the magazine girl has a scowl on her face. The energy you embody is far more important than the clothes you wear, this is so important to learn. Let's really break down the traits of feminine energy.

Firstly, there is nurturing. Some misconceptions with nurturing is that people think this means mothering which it does not, nurturing means you are going to nurture the behavior you want to see, or encourage the behavior you want to see, so in turn you see more of it. This is a very powerful trait of feminine energy and extremely effective. This is also a way of managing expectations, such as a woman could say - I would love it if you took me on a date this Friday. In that sentence she is nurturing the behavior she wants to see and managing her expectations in her feminine energy. The opposite of that is if she said - you haven't taken me on a date in ages. See with feminine energy it is always positive. Then after the date she would say - thank you so much, you are a fantastic partner. More nurturing the behavior she wants to see. This sounds super simple yer, unfortunately most women never do it, it's so easy. Nurture the behavior you want to see and you will be seeing way more of it. Most people constantly critique behaviors in a relationship never encourage the good behaviors, this is not an effective method of teaching people how to have relationships with us. If you properly nurture the behavior you want to see then you won't need to punish bad behavior, the bad stuff will automatically fade away. For lack of a better example this is very similar to training dogs, when a dog does the right thing he is rewarded, constantly rewarding the good behavior then eventually that is all you will see. Humans are family similar. So remember before you start talking, take a second and ask yourself if you are talking in your feminine energy or are you being counter productive.

The second trait is caring caring, with a woman in her feminine energy you can tell she truly cares, it's not superficial with her, she deeply cares. She cares about you, your goals, your success, she wants to succeed, she is your ultimate cheerleader, she cares deeply about her partner and her family. Some women fall out of their feminine energy and fall into a rut of not caring at all, this is mainly due to environment. If a woman's environment is bad or negative or unsafe then she will not be in her feminine energy and she will be forced into her masculine energy in order to protect herself and survive. As a woman it is hard to remain in your feminine energy at all times but you can be very selective with your environment and who is in it. One of the most important skills for women to learn is who to allow into your life, if you allow the wrong people into your life, your life will get really bad really fast. Be extremely selective only to let positive influences in, if you have a healthy environment and good people around you then it will be easy to step into your feminine energy and be very caring.

Third trait is supportive and my favorite one, my wife embodies this trait perfectly, I knew before I met her that I needed a wife who was super supportive of my goals and would help me achieve them, most women would complain I work too much, if you are a man reading this and you are super ambitious like me and most likely want to work 24/7 then you need a wife who will work alongside you and help you build something great, not one that sits on the side lines complaining you don't spend enough time together. I'll tell my wife my goals and she says - why stop there? Why not aim higher?

I love that, that really embodies supportive well, I truly believe this is where the quote comes from - behind every successful man is a smart woman. I wouldn't be 10% as successful as I am today without my wife, she has made me so successful. It's crazy, no way I could do all this myself. Remember fella's, the wrong woman will make you broke, the right woman will make you rich, and it all comes down to support, is she willing to be in the trenches with you, putting in the hard work, the 110% effort 100 hours a week. My dad would've been 10 times more successful if my mum was supportive but she wasn't, she never really learnt how to be feminine unfortunately. My wife is super supportive and super strong, two traits I need in a wife. She is truly amazing.

The fourth trait of femininity is joyous, the lovely trait. This basically means to have a good attitude and a sunny disposition. Life can seem gray, overcast, overall stressful and bitter, a woman's job is to be a man's joy. His ray of sunshine in an otherwise cloudy world, a joyous happy woman is so attractive, you are pulled to her, you want to talk to her, you want to be around her. Unfortunately many women have what society so crudely calls resting bitch face, or a face like a cat's asshole, that term is pretty funny but it does fit many women. As a woman if you're walking around super serious with a scowl on your face no one is going to like you, fix your face. Regardless of how good looking you think you are, no one wants to be around a bitter cynical woman, you must embrace and really let that joyous energy shine, more people will like you and the more you will like yourself as well. Some of you may be asking, how can I be joyous? It's not overly complicated, one of the best ways to do this is to smile, put a big smile on your face and just keep smiling, pass someone on the street? Smile! At the checkout counter at the shops? Smile! Smile everywhere, let your smile shine bright, you will notice other people around you will smile more, it can be beautifully infectious. Another way you can be more joyous is by intentionally choosing the right words, we have all been around people sometimes and all they do is whinge and complain! So annoying! In your joyous energy you are going to be saying lots of things you're grateful for, how lucky we are, how beautiful the weather is, lots and lots of positive uplifting statements, this in turn will make you feel better and those around you will feel more positive as well. This all plays into emotional regulation, if you can intentionally choose the emotions you want to feel then your life is going to be so much better, intentionally choose to be happy, choose to be joyous, choose to be enthusiastic.

Feminine energy is so powerful, when embodied properly people around you will feel better. A feminine woman is like the soul food of people, it feels good for your soul to be around that person. If a woman is in her feminine energy and she leaves someone's home, everyone in that home feels great, uplifted and overall better for the experience. If a woman is in her masculine energy then everything just feels off, a woman in her masculine energy makes everyone nervous, uneasy, uncomfortable. I'm sure many of you have experienced this first hand and seen it in others. When someone isn't in their correct energy everything feels off, you can tell they aren't happy within themselves, nor their environment. Whatever environment you're in, if people there aren't in their correct energies then it just feels weird, it doesn't feel right. In life we can't control many environments but we can control our own home, does your home feel right? Does everyone there properly embody their energies? If they do, the house will feel truly like a home, if the people there don't embody their energy properly then it will feel uncomfortable.

As you know now masculine and feminine energy is truly a powerful super power, one you can embody which can drastically improve your life, unfortunately there is many forms of kryptonite that can weaken this superpower of yours, one of those is your environment,

We live in a time in history where society tells us that it is okay that a man is feminine and a female is masculine, and we wonder why we are having trouble with relationships. I coach couple after couple and person after person that suffers from the same problem: the man doesn't know how to be masculine and the woman is acting like the man.

Ladies, this isn't your fault, because if your man was acting truly masculine, you would automatically want to be in your feminine energy. I like to think of it as a see-saw, or scales; when one side goes up the other side goes down, and vice versa. So as time goes by in a relationship and the man starts acting more feminine, the female has no choice; her masculine energy automatically goes up, and she cannot control it.

Masculine and Feminine energy is very important. The way I describe it is simple: I want men to embody masculine energy, the traits of which include leadership, ambition, decisiveness, and protection. I want women to embody feminine energy which includes nurturing, caring, supportive, and joyous.

Here's something to remember about these beautiful brains we have: even though we are living in the twentieth century, our brain is the same as it was 100,000 years ago, and our hormones are the same. Basically, we haven't changed a lot, so women are still attracted to tall, strong, masculine males— because 100,000 years ago they wanted to find a partner to breed with who was strong enough to protect the tribe, pro- tect the family, and lead both to success and prosperity. We haven't changed that much from our ancestors. Women still want a strong confident alpha male leader, and men still want a beautiful feminine woman. You can't argue with nature; a lot of people try and it always ends badly. It is far easier to work with nature.

In his book *The Way of the Superior Man*, author David Deida describes feminine energy like the ocean. It is:

- Vast
- Directionless
- Either calm or violent
- Beautiful

On the flip side, masculine energy is like a river in that it:

- Goes in one direction, toward its purpose
- Is passionate and motivated
- Will not stop until it reaches its goal
- Cannot be stopped when it is raging

It is extremely important to understand masculine and feminine energy in-depth, because it consumes everything we do. The more you understand it, the better your life will become.

There are a whole bunch of things men do which slowly puts them into their feminine energy and lowers the attraction level of the female. Men often attract what they fear, so they might fear their lady will leave them, or cheat on them. By living in fear, they become so focused on the fear that they automatically start acting needy and desperate in an attempt to not let their fears come true. Unfortunately, by acting needy and desperate, their fears end up coming true.

Guys, you truly need to be fearless; that's what being a strong confident alpha male leader is all about. If you fear your lady will leave you, say to yourself, "Pfft, who cares? There are mil- lions of attractive women and I'm a catch. I'm not afraid of losing her." If you truly believe that, then you won't ever act in your feminine energy, and her attraction will stay high.

Communication plays a large role in the different energies. So something to remember is that women speak out of emotion and men speak out of logic.

What does that mean? It means that sometimes a female will say something and it isn't fact. Rather, she is communicating how she feels at that moment. So you two may be an amazing couple, and you have done everything perfectly the first year you are together, then you both have an off day and she says you are a terrible partner. It's not a fact. You are actually an amazing partner; she is simply telling you how she is feeling at that moment. So don't take it personally; that is the time to communicate more and talk it out. We will talk more about that in the communication chapters.

Girls, there are many techniques to keep you in your feminine energy, such as spending time with other feminine women or watching feminine women on social media or TV. Remember the content we consume is ultimately what we become.

Always try to communicate in a feminine way. If he feels criticised by what you said, then you most likely said it in a masculine way, not a feminine way. Say you really want your man to wash the dishes. You could say, "Geez you're lazy, why don't you do the dishes?" Or you could walk up to him, slowly slide your fingertips up and down his arms while looking up into his eyes and say in a nice, feminine tone, "Could you please do the dishes for me, handsome?"

Which one sounds better? Life gets a lot easier if you communicate in a feminine way and you are in your feminine energy. If you are truly in your feminine energy and he is truly in his masculine energy, then you will never have any arguments.

Feminine energy is like a rose: big, beautiful, it attracts the bees, and is soft. But a rose also has thorns; a lot of women lead with their thorns and not with their flower and wonder why they have so much trouble. The thorns are there for life-and- death situations, nothing more. Girls, practice always leading with your rose. It's impossible to get angry and argue with a big beautiful soft rose, but it is very easy to argue with thorns.

Feminine energy at its core is sensitive because it feels more and a lot deeper than masculine energy and should be protected. Feminine energy is also patient, not aggressive, and it is happy to wait for what it wants. It is also caring. It cares deeply for the others in its family and tribe, and even if they hurt it, it cares about things on a much deeper level than masculine energy does. A very natural feminine state is one of nurturing; it is in its nature to nurture and mother its young. It is a truly beau- tiful thing, very caring and nurturing of babies and young to see them be happy and survive. A beautiful mother with her newborn baby is one of the most beautiful things in the world.

Feminine energy is also gentle. It doesn't like being boisterous, it likes to be touched softly and gently. It is also emotional, and feminine emotion can go up and down quite quickly and regularly. I'm sure we have all seen this, and even though sometimes it can be challenging and frustrating, accept it for what it is and try to enjoy it. Remember, the sea can be rough.

And of course feminine energy is loving, a very deep feeling that cares a lot about inclusiveness and love; if it doesn't feel loved then it will feel drained.

There is a lot to feminine energy; however, it is truly a beautiful thing. Unfortunately, so many women are in their masculine energy the majority of the time because they have surrounded themselves with weak, soft men. This in turn makes the woman into the alpha male, and she can never enjoy her femininity. Then she often wonders why all her relationships are struggling, and when she does find an attractive guy, they seem to argue a lot.

Be very conscious of this and really make the effort to be in your feminine energy. You have to make a conscious effort to be in your feminine energy; it won't just happen naturally unless you are around a truly strong, confident alpha male leader. Also be aware that you can use your feminine energy to make a man more masculine. The first trait of feminine energy is nurturing. You nurture the behaviour you want to see, so don't give a man a shoulder to cry on, because this only makes him weaker. Instead, be his cheerleader. Tell him he is smart, strong, and can solve any problem—this is how you push a man into his masculinity.

Now masculine energy is obviously much different than feminine energy. There have been a lot of extremely masculine tribes and groups over the years, such as the Spartan warriors who were very masculine because they were forced to be that way, and they trained very hard from a very young age.

Unfortunately, it seems that the harder the times a boy goes through, the tougher of a man he becomes, and even more sad is the fact that we want to make our boys' lives very easy and soft, so the majority of boys just sit around playing Xbox or computer games and eat junk food. We wonder why they have no discipline or motivation, but discipline and motivation aren't traits you are born with; they are built, trained and learnt skills, just like driving or fighting. You aren't born knowing how to drive; you have to learn how. Similarly, discipline is a muscle that must be trained and built. You can read a lot about push- ups but it won't make you good at them, and the same goes for discipline and motivation.

This is how I stay disciplined and motivated: I wake up every morning at 4:30 am and drive to the beach, do my priming and gratitude exercises, and go for a cold-water dawn swim. I did that routine for a long time but then I decided to make it more challenging. I built my own ice bath, which is just a chest freezer waterproofed and filled up. Then I turn it on and have ice water. So now every morning I jump into that for six minutes. I'm not sure why I chose six minutes, but I never tried any other time. I just set my timer for that long and never changed it.

No, it's not easy, it's hard work. If it were easy, it wouldn't build up my discipline and motivation. Discipline is a muscle that needs to be trained. Cold water swims and priming builds it for me, so find your thing. If you're a man who truly wants to step into his masculine energy, then you need to embrace leadership, ambition, decisiveness, and protection. So start with your goals, write a long list of at least twenty goals, work aggressively on them, and be patient with results.

I'm coaching one couple, whom we will call Fred and Mary. Mary has had a very hard childhood and life so far; she has had to pretty much raise herself and care for herself. She never had much help, and this consequently made her into a very masculine female. She's had to be masculine to survive, but unfortunately now she is in a relationship with Fred and they have kids together and they constantly butt heads because they are both trying to be masculine.

Their relationship is now a 10/10 because I kept working with her to get her into her feminine energy and gave her techniques on how to stay in it. I talked to her several times about nurturing her rose. Feminine energy is not just for romantic relationships. A woman can be in her feminine energy around her friends, family, and co-workers too. Just be nice! Relax and nurture the behaviour in others you want to see.

One of the main things I taught Fred is how to stay emotionally stable. He would get quite angry and emotional when she was testing him, and the arguments got very nasty. If you are the leader and you are in your masculine energy, you must remain emotionally stable; if you lose your temper when she is testing you, then you have failed the test. Women test to see how strong you are, and if you get all emotional then she will see that you aren't that strong and her attraction will keep going down.

So with Fred now mastering his emotions and remaining emotionally stable, the relationship has flourished and become a 10/10.

Feminine energy spends a lot of time testing. A woman is constantly testing her man in different ways. Guys, if you think your girl is trying to piss you off or get under your skin on purpose, she's testing you. And girls, you may be trying to annoy him, and not even realise you are doing it. A lot of females test and don't realise because they do it on a subconscious level.

The reason women test men is because of safety. Remember the brain we have is thousands of years old, and thousands of years ago a woman would test a man to see if he was strong enough and worthy to breed with. It still happens today and always will happen; that is just the way humans are. The thought pattern that goes through a female's mind is, "Well, if he gets really upset when I annoy him, then how will he handle what life is going to throw at him? How is he going to provide for and protect us? That is why women test, and guys, you need to pass these tests. Every time you fail a test, her attraction for you goes down, and every time you pass, her attraction for you increases.

So be very aware that all women test; however, the higher her attraction is for you, then the less she will test, so if her attraction for you is already a 10/10, then she will barely test at all, and the test will be very easy to pass.

If her attraction for you is a 5/10, then she will test you a lot, and the tests will be very hard. She is pretty much seeing if she can break you, and she is testing your strength and your masculinity. Women want a guy who is extremely strong and can't be broken.

Masculine and Feminine energy also play a massive role in parenting. Feminine energy is naturally caring and nurturing while masculine energy is strong and aggressive. That's why you may find that kids instinctively listen to their fathers or males more than their mothers or females.

A lot of women try to discipline the same way a man does but it doesn't work, and they find themselves going deep into their masculine energy to get their kids to listen, but this is really bad, and they are becoming something they really don't want to be anyway. You may remember from school a strong confident male teacher whom everyone just listened to, and he didn't even need to raise his voice. Everyone would just listen, because he was an alpha male.

Ladies, don't try to be an alpha male. You can't fight nature, so you need to approach it differently. Approach it femininely; make people and kids want to be your friend so they are trying to get your validation. Kids won't fear their mothers or a female teacher like they do a male, but if the female acts in the right way, they will want her acceptance and validation; this is your power. Use it to your advantage.

Men, be aware that when you are being a strong, confident alpha male leader, you may scare children. Doing so will make their mothers upset. If you try using strong discipline, the mother may feel like you are bullying the child or something like that. This is extremely common, but don't get deterred. The mother or female needs to understand that men and women parent differently, and they need to respect the process of discipline. You need to be hard on kids so they grow up strong and resilient. If you are too soft on them, they will grow up weak and bratty, which is terrible and a real disservice to the child.

A lot of people alive today were raised wrong, resulting in them being weak. Consequently, they have trouble doing even the simplest tasks. Men, be hard on your children and explain to their mothers that it's for their own good and that they need to support you during this time or go into another room.

Personally, I've been teaching my kids martial arts, mainly karate and jujitsu since they could walk. This was a great way for me to personally teach them respect and discipline. Their mother was not allowed in the room while we trained, and no other female was allowed in if they were going to hinder training. If someone was to slow us down or complain we were training too hard, then they would not be allowed in. Men, this is the approach you need to take, and your children will turn out much better if you are hard on them. This approach can differ slightly depending on whether your child is a girl or a boy.

I personally don't believe in the term "toxic masculinity" because if a man is being a bully, being violent, involved in domestic violence or anything similar, then he isn't being mas- culine. Masculinity is protective by nature, so if a man is beating his wife, then he isn't protecting her, so he can't be being mas- culine. He is simply being weak and is full of insecurities and weakness resulting in him being a bully. Disciplining a child has the purpose and goal of making that child more successful in that particular area. Bullying them is the opposite goal. Bullying is not okay and will hinder the child's success. To clarify, discipline versus bullying is about intention; other than that, just try your best.

Society seems to have filled the word masculinity with negativity, teaching people it's bad to be masculine and that men should be more feminine. The majority of men are already too feminine; that is why so many relationships are ending prematurely. So many women contact me saying their man isn't acting like a man, and he needs to "man up" and all sorts of stuff. Men being feminine is not the answer to your prob- lems; it's the cause. Women, being masculine, being in charge, and leading is okay in the workplace but not in your romantic relationships. In that case, you are leading with your thorns and just hurting yourself.

Every single man strives to be a strong, confident alpha male leader.

Every single woman should strive to be a beautiful, feminine, sweet and caring lady.

A few people disagree with me on this, but I truly don't care what your current energy is like. Guys, if you think you are just naturally feminine and you should be happy with that, stop it! You aren't just naturally feminine, your weak pathetic environment and parents have made you this way, and you should say to them, "Fuck you for making me into a little bitch." They did you a disservice and you are going to have to work hard to become a strong, confident alpha male leader. No one is born that way; you have to work at it.

Women, if you think you like being a strong, confident alpha leader in all environments, then that's why your relationship is shit. Feminine energy in its natural state is to surrender. If you want to be the leader, go and play sports. At home, you have to encourage your man to lead.

When the woman is the leader in the relationship, then you start hearing them say sentences like, "Oh, me and my child are coming," or "I have three kids" when they only have two. By not being a leader, guys, you become one of her children, and it's pathetic.

Guys, never say the sentence, "I just have to check with the boss first," referring to your wife. What a weak, pathetic sentence to say. Might as well say, "Oh, I just have to check with mommy before saying yes." Be the leader, make a decision. Don't ask permission. People act like this and wonder why the attraction in their relationship is declining.

I often hear women say, "I don't want to be led, I don't need a leader, a relationship should be 50/50." It's all rubbish. If you have some negative beliefs around leadership, it is because you don't know what a leader is.

A leader in the relationship wants to lead the relationship to success, wants the best for you and the relationship, wants to protect it and ensure its survival, and works hard to ensure it is constantly improving. Being a leader is only a good thing; there is not a single negative thing about leadership. All men should try to embody as many leadership traits as possible. Girls may say they don't need a leader, but deep down, they want you to take their hand and lead the way.

Although some of you believe a relationship should be 50/50, it is more like 70/30. Because the man has to be the leader, and the leader is responsible for everything, that makes his responsibil- ity for the relationship far higher than the female, so it should be at 70/30. If the relationship is at 50/50 then the man isn't being the leader, and the woman is starting to lead, and trouble can start to arise. Remember life isn't fair and relationships aren't fair, so get that shit out of your head. Trouble only arises when you start fighting nature. Stop fighting it and let it flow.

As you can see, masculine and feminine energy go into every single facet of everything we do. Men, embody those mascu- line traits; and females, embody those feminine traits, and your relationship will improve a lot and you'll be a lot happier.

Leadership

So you may be asking yourself, "How does leadership affect me and my relationship?" It affects your relationship greatly and everyone should be striving to be the best leader they can be. John C. Maxwell said, "The measure of a leader is not the number of people who serve him but the number of people he serves." Amazing statement. How many leaders have you created?

At this point you may be asking yourself, "So doesn't someone have to always wear the pants in the relationship and be the boss?" Firstly, I hate the word boss. A leader and a boss are very different things. A leader wants what's best for his team, whereas a boss wants what's best for himself. So a leader in the relationship wants to lead the relationship and family to success.

Leadership and masculine energy are closely tied together. I know it sounds sexist; however, it is a man's job to lead his relationship and family to success. Men are supposed to be the leaders. Many people are triggered by this, but it is just nature and how we are, so don't fight it; just accept it.

Many women strive to be the leader at home; they want to be

the alpha male. These types of relationships where the woman is the leader never make it to a 10/10. All the couples who come to me for help meet this criteria; the women are masculine and the men are feminine, and the woman is the leader making all the decisions and calling all the shots. Their relationship is terrible and in a lot of trouble, and they know it.

One of the first things I do with couples like this is teach them about masculine and feminine energy and teach the female that femininity is to surrender. Femininity is a lover not a fighter, while masculinity is a fighter and is never to surrender. That's why masculinity is so closely tied to leadership. All the women I coach find it very difficult to let go of this power they have and to step back from being the leader and letting their men lead, but they get there eventually with enough coaching and their men stepping up.

A king will have trouble leading if his queen doesn't support him. One of the main reasons these men have such trouble being the leader is because their wives are complete bitches who hold them back from leading and the men are too weak to do anything about it. Guys, no matter how strong, mean, or angry your wife is, don't let her lead, don't let her make all the decisions, and don't let her be the ruler. You are the king of your castle.

Guys, I have a secret for you: Women don't want to be the leaders anyway. They don't want to be masculine; they don't want to be a ball-busting bitch. They are this way because they feel they have to be to survive. No woman is ever masculine with me because they know they can't get their way with me; they know straight away they can't lead me, because I am too strong, too masculine, too certain, and too confident. Guys, you need to have so much strength that no woman will see you as a doormat. They won't try to argue with you because you will never surrender. You need to show unbreakable strength and emotional stability. No matter what anyone says they can't stop you from achieving your goals, and anything in the way of you achieving your goals will be smashed.

Watching author and coach Tony Robbins talk to a masculine woman is very funny. No matter how tough she tries to be, if she comes to him with a masculine bitchy attitude, she gets nowhere fast. He is super hard on her until she usually ends up crying and in her feminine energy. A truly strong, confident alpha male leader will never surrender. He will always lead and his strength will be unbreakable. Guys, you need to adopt this and use it in every single thing you do in life: your relationship, business, gym, and family. Be a leader everywhere and always strive for success.

Girls, there is a lot you can do in this department as well; it's called supporting your king. If he makes a decision then back him, stand by his side, and support his decision. It doesn't matter if it's a bad decision; support him anyway, and let him lead.

Many women are not supportive of their husbands. He will have an idea or make a decision and his wife will complain or disagree and want to argue, making him second guess himself. He will get insecure with his decision and the wife will get her way. But if you do this long enough, the relationship will end. Girls, if you are reading this you may be thinking, "Well some- times my way is best and I'm smarter than he is." However, that is the type of attitude that ends in divorce. So do you want to be right, or do you want to be happy? And thinking you are right all the time is so arrogant; just support your husband and be happy he made a decision. Let go of the reins.

One of my female clients asked me, "Can it be 50/50?"

Now, if you think about it, that sentence is a masculine sentence. She is fighting for every bit of power she can have. Instead of being feminine, enjoying her life, and being a good mother, she is trying to hold on to as much control as possible. Relationships aren't 50/50. They are 80/20 because the man is responsible for the relationship, he is the leader, and all the responsibility falls on his shoulders. Ladies, this isn't a bad thing. Enjoy not having to be the leader. You can sit back, enjoy your life, and enjoy being the joy and love in his life. You don't need to be tough or discipline anyone, and you can get every single thing in life you can possibly want using your femininity anyway. You don't need to be the leader.

Think about it like this: imagine you have a punch card and there are ten spots on the card. You only get the one card for your entire life, and each spot is for arguments, so you only get ten arguments for your entire life. How are you going to spend them? Are you going to argue every night with your partner and have the same argument again and again, going around in circles? Or will you learn effective communication and learn how to solve the issue and get your relationship to a 10/10?

Why can't there be two leaders? Are there ever two chefs in a kitchen? I'm not sure since I've never worked in a kitchen, but there is always one person making the final decisions. Other people can weigh in on the decisions but only that one person can make the final call. Some women have a lot of trouble letting go of power, and it is very sad to see. You can't both lead. One person needs to surrender sometimes. It is feminine to surrender, and it isn't a bad thing, girls.

Unfortunately, statistically, if a woman is the leader in the relationship, the relationship will fail. I have seen this many many times. I wish it wasn't true, but it is. I know it sounds sexist, blah blah blah. I've heard it all before, but I have been coaching people in the art of relationships for years. When the woman leads, it fails. That is a fact! So, girls, stop trying to lead.

More importantly, guys, stop being so fucking weak that your girl has to lead. You're a fucking man! Stop acting like a boy and let me hear you roar like a fucking lion! Like a Spartan soldier! You are in this mess because you are so fucking weak, and your girl thinks she needs to lead because you can't do it! Because you are pathetic! That's why you're reading a relation- ship book instead of getting a blow job right now! You see those guys who are really mean to their wives, talk to them like shit, and somehow their relationship is great and for some reason their wives love them to death, and you think to yourself, "But he's so mean." The girl sees it as mean, too, but she also sees the meanness as strength. All women want a strong, confident alpha male leader.

Sometimes a leader's job is to let the people he is leading make decisions. Think about a company. The big manager doesn't stand over your shoulder and tell you how to type, does he? Because that would be called micro-management, and that is not leadership. Sometimes being a leader means letting someone makes mistakes. Even though you know what they are doing is going to turn out badly, you let them do it anyway, because making a mistake is one of the best ways to learn. That is called leading from the back. There are many different ways to lead.

Also realise that being a control freak is far different than being a good leader. A good leader isn't a control freak at all, and sometimes a good leader doesn't seem like they are leading at all. A truly great leader can almost lead in a secret way. They know how to influence and make you perform better, such as leading by example. Although this isn't really direct leading, it can be very powerful. Remember that idea and look into it if you have to because it's a good one.

So to clarify, girls, if your man is a good leader he will try to turn you into a leader as well. Not to lead the relationship but to take responsibility for your own life and lead other people in your life and your business or work to success. He will build you up and make you feel emotionally safe and secure. You will love to confide in him because he is a great source of strength you can draw from. Keep that in mind guys; women come to us for strength. We don't go to them for strength. See the difference? After that paragraph it doesn't sound so bad, does it? Having a leader in your life is only a positive, never ever a negative. If you see it as a negative, it means they aren't a leader or you have such a massive ego you think you are God and you hate anyone having more power than you.

A good leader doesn't oppress you, and doesn't bully. A good leader builds you up and fills you with a feeling of emotional safety so you can feel confident. They want what's best for you and they want to see you succeed. Having a leader in your life is a fantastic blessing, and if there is someone in your life who is like this, then thank them because most people in the world don't have something like this in their lives.

Guys, if the relationship is going bad, you need to take ownership, and if something goes wrong you need to take ownership. If your girl says, "That's your fault," you need to say "Yes, it was." Take full responsibility! Don't argue with someone if they are blaming you for something. Instead, thank them for giving you the power or responsibility, since they are giving you ownership of the situation. I consider that a wonderful gift. But guys, there is a flip side to that coin as well. Enjoy taking responsibility for every single thing in your life but never ever give it away, never blame someone else saying, "It's his or her fault I don't have this or haven't done that." That is not something a leader does. A good leader always takes 100 percent of the responsibility and never ever blames anyone else.

Be the architect of your own life, don't just be reactive. Most people are just running around reacting to things. Take ownership and take control. Remember, you are in charge of your own life; no one else can design your life for you. However, a good leader can help others design their own lives. Who have you helped lately? Have you helped someone else become a leader lately?

PART II

Attraction

Attraction

In life and relationships attraction is everything. I really can't stress enough how important attraction is. In fact, it is so important that it is an important pillar in achieving a 10/10 relationship.

Now, what do I mean by "attraction"? How pretty someone is? Not exactly. When I say attraction, I mean their entire energy, personality, looks—everything. You may be able to remember a time when someone walked into a room and everyone looked at them, males and females. That person who everyone looked at has a high attraction level. Everyone wants to talk to that person, and it doesn't have anything to do with sex.

No one is born with this trait; it must be learnt, just like everything in dating and relationships.

In the past I was terrible with relationships. I experienced heartbreak after heartbreak, with no idea what I was doing. I didn't have any desire to learn about relationships until my last relationship. It was devastating, and I dreaded going home each day after work. It got to the point where I was severely depressed and suicidal. I had no idea how to build attraction and embrace masculinity effectively, and the worst part is I was with the wrong person. Even though I had a wonderful son with that woman ten years earlier and tried to make it work, it was absolutely impossible. For those who try to stay together for the kids, you are wasting your time. If someone isn't your ideal partner then end it quickly and move on—life is short.

That was the point I said to myself, "The past was bad, the present is bad, and the future will be bad unless I do some- thing about it now." Upon making that decision, I ended that relationship and started on my personal development journey. I learned the power of attraction so that you can too.

Now back to attraction. As I said, it is extremely important to be constantly judging your partner's attraction for you. There are several ways to do this.

Imagine something I call an attraction meter. From 1–10, if someone's attraction for you is at a 1, then they despise you and want you to die; they have nothing for you but pure hatred. And at the other end of the scale, you have 10. If someone's attraction for you is at a 10, they will constantly tell you how much they love you and want to marry you, and they will be buying you gifts and constantly touching you. They are madly in love with you, and this is what you want to achieve.

Something to remember with attraction is, everything you say and do makes your partner's attraction for you go up or down, regardless if you're in an "exclusive" relationship or not.

We always want to increase our partner's attraction to us, and if you're single you want to try to become what you want to attract.

What does that mean? If you want someone with an amazing body, ripped abs and all that, but you are a fat slob who loves Netflix and Xbox, then you are going to have trouble attracting that person. If you want someone who is a 10/10, then you need to become a 10/10 too. And throughout your entire life, you should be constantly trying to improve yourself. Even if your partner's attraction for you is at a 10/10, you should always be trying to improve.

Regarding attraction and dating for guys, if a female says "yes" to going on a date with you, her attraction for you is at least a 5/10. If it is under a five, then she won't go out with you. It's your job to date her properly so her attraction goes up to a 9 or a 10. A lot of guys don't get a second date with a girl because they lowered her attraction on the date, instead of raising it. The first date is so crucial in getting that attraction up if you ever want a second. Another mistake most people make is the way they communicate before, during, and after the date, because this can turn the other person off so much that they will never talk to the other person again. I will talk about the perfect date in a later chapter.

A lot of guys come to me who have been married for ten or twenty years and tell me that their wife has just left them and wants a divorce, and they proceed to tell me that they thought they did everything right for the first nineteen years, but in the twentieth year things started to go south. This makes me laugh, since they are literally blind to the slow death of the relationship. They don't understand why the relationship died or how. They didn't notice the slow decline in attraction.

It is vital you constantly judge your partner's level of attraction for you, because once it gets down to a 5/10, then break-ups happen. If your partner's attraction for you is a 9 or 10/10, then they will never leave you, and they will do anything to keep you in their life. I also hear a lot of excuses from guys, like "Oh, she lives too far away and it will never work." The rule of attraction trumps all excuses and reasons. If you can get a girl's attraction for you to a 10/10, she will leave her family, religion, country, and everything to be with you. The only reason you can't get the relationship to work is because you failed in getting the attraction to a high enough level.

MEASURING ATTRACTION

I've already said several times you must be constantly measuring your partner's attraction, but how do you do that?

Some quick questions you need to ask yourself are:

- How often are they touching me? (It doesn't need to be sexual touching.)
- How often are you having sex?
- When was the last time they bought you a gift?
- When was the last date?
- Do they listen to what you have to say?
- Do they go out of their way for you? (Doing things they might not really want to do, such as chores or cleaning for you, or giving you a blowjob or taking care of you when you don't feel 100 percent.)
- Do they desire to please you?
- Do they value your opinion?
- Do they respect you?
- And lastly, something you should do is once in a while, maybe monthly, ask your partner straight out, what would you rate our relationship out of 10?
-

It is very important you ask the question like that. They aren't rating you; they're rating the relationship. Then let's say they reply, "Um, maybe a 7/10." You must then ask, "Why a seven? And how can we get it to a 10/10?" Then they will tell you exactly what they want.

If you aren't constantly measuring your partner's attraction for you, that's when things slowly slip down and down until you are fighting a lot and looking at breaking up. It's very easy to be complacent with your relationship, especially if you are an entrepreneur or just a very busy person.

I often fall into this trap because I am very passionate about my purpose in life. I sometimes tend to forget about my beautiful partner because I work all the time, every day. However, I am very good at measuring my partner's attraction for me, so I can tell as soon as it starts slipping downward that I need to do something, which usually means I have to put my phone away and spend some quality one-on-one time with her.

If you aren't the best communicator and your partner isn't very good at expressing their feelings in a constructive manner and neither of you measure the attraction, then the relationship will be difficult. If this is you, then study this book over and over so you learn how to build attraction and effectively communicate so you can get your relationship to a 10/10.

So the takeaway points to remember from this chapter are:

- Always be measuring your partner's attraction.
- Try to get their attraction for you to a 10/10.
- Become what you want to attract.
-

- Even if the attraction is a 10/10, keep trying to improve.
- Attraction is everything.

Some people talk about love and lust. These are hard to measure and hard to describe. What is easy to measure is attraction, because you can't fake attraction and you can't hide it. Once you start looking for it and seeing the signs, it is very easy to see and measure and use to your advantage. So I'm hoping after you finish reading this chapter that you start measuring everyone's attraction for you and start working on ways to increase your own attractive qualities.

PART III

Courtship

Ideal Partner

Finding your ideal partner is very important. Unfortunately most people don't put much effort into finding their ideal partner. Most people pick their partners from proximity and attraction. Just because someone lives near you and is pretty isn't a good reason to marry them; it is a lot more complicated than that. If you want to find someone who you want to spend the rest of your life with, be picky.

Society tells us that being picky is bad, and we shouldn't be so picky in life. I'm telling you the exact opposite: be as picky as possible when choosing a partner. If you can walk away, then do it. If you can't walk away even if you wanted to, then they may be the one.

The first step in the task of finding your ideal partner is to make a list. A very long, detailed list. Imagine it is the year 3000 and you can put your list into a computer and your dream partner jumps out with the looks, the personality, the hobbies, the job, everything which makes them them.

So take out your notepad now and write your ideal list; it should have on there:

- Their height
- Hair colour
- Eye colour
- Weight
- Size
- Body shape
- Personality
- Hobbies
- Career
- Family
- Goals
- Ambitions

You get the point—it needs to be very long and detailed. At the end of this list, I want you to also write a list of ten red flags. The reason for this exercise is because many people get overwhelmed with emotion and their emotions mask the red flags. One of your red flags may be smoking. Then you meet a person who smokes, and you say to yourself, "Well, they smoke but they are really nice so I'll ignore it or try to make them quit." Bad idea. Don't go into a relationship wanting to change everything about the person. Choose a partner you are happy with from the start.

Just making this list and reading it at least once a week will be very profitable for you. The universe will start showing you people who match most of the things on your list. It is the law of attraction: write it down and it is 80 percent more likely to come true.

It is hard to find something if you don't know what you are looking for. A lot of people say they want to find a partner but have no idea what sort, or anything about them. If you want to go for a drive but have no idea where you are going, then you will just end up going in circles.

A lot of people tend to do this; it is quite a vicious cycle actu- ally. You meet an attractive partner, then it turns out they are too different to get along with and you break up, resulting in your self-esteem declining. You say to yourself that you will be alone forever and should settle for anyone. That is why so many people are in relationships with people they shouldn't be in relationships with. Instead, ask the universe for what you want and it will deliver. Be as picky as possible.

I've had clients sign up to my program, and they have been single for years (some for decades) and have no idea how to get a partner and even whether or not anyone wants them. Within one month of signing up with me, they find their ideal partner. I am constantly amazed by this. If you just say yes to yourself and put out into the universe what you want, the universe will hand it to you on a silver platter. I love it. One of my clients, Emma, came to me single and after writing out very clearly what she wanted and starting to put that out and put herself out there too, James walked into her life soon after, and they now have a fantastic 10/10 relationship.

If you meet someone and go on a few dates, and you can walk away, do it. If you feel like you could walk away without caring, then that person isn't the one. Be as picky as possible. This is someone you may spend the rest of your life with.

Some people run into trouble with someone who speaks the opposite love language than them. Knowing your partner's love language will give you a good idea on how to make them feel the most loved. If you really love cuddling and are a very affection- ate person, don't get into a relationship with someone who hates it; otherwise, you will be left feeling sad, lonely, and unloved.

It's extremely important to know what you want and just as important to know about yourself as well. Knowing oneself is of paramount importance in all aspects of life. After you find your ideal partner, you need to know how to communicate and date properly because you may find that amazing person, then you stuff it up by acting stupid on the first date, and they never call you again. I will go through dating thoroughly in the next chapter.

Remember, there are billions of people on the earth, so be picky. If the person has too many red flags, let them go; it is better for both of you. Once doing this list, you will be surprised at how fast people who match your list start showing up. It is the universe giving you opportunities, and it is up to you not to waste them.

You may look back on your life up to this point and see all the past relationships you have had, and why each one of your past partners weren't your ideal partner. If you are anything like me, you may slap yourself in the face a few times and say, "What was I thinking?" I have done that many times. Don't be too hard on yourself. If those other relationships didn't happen, then you wouldn't be the person you are today.

Remember in the chapter about attraction and becoming what you want to attract? I hope you have started improving yourself, because if your ideal partner's list is someone with a 10/10 body and you are a fat slob who is addicted to TV, then the universe will laugh at you. It needs to be realistic. So start improving yourself and keep improving yourself forever. Keep learning and never stop. Everyone loves ambitious people; nobody likes a loser who has no goals or drive. I have seen quite a few times now, two people with two different ideal partner lists come together, and they were everything on each other's list. What are the chances? Quite slim I would've guessed, but it happens all the time. The universe makes it happen. You just need to have an open mind and an open heart.

Try to imagine what your ideal partner's list would look like, and what you think is on that list. This will drastically increase your chances of being with that person, and it will be a lot easier.

Something to always remember is that dating should be easy, so if you meet someone and dating them is really hard and pain- ful, then they are the wrong person for you. It should be easy and enjoyable; both parties should want to see each other all the time. Some people believe this is far-fetched and not really possible, but if you say no to the wrong people and only let your true, ideal partner in, then it will be easy, smooth, and natural.

Often you may meet someone and you are texting each other a lot, and then they are taking longer and longer to respond each time, until they start ghosting you for days at a time, really showing that their interest isn't that high. Dating your ideal partner should not be like that. Rather, they should want to message you heaps, talk to you constantly, and be around you constantly. If they constantly have an excuse not to see you and only make time to see you once a week or even less than that, then they aren't your ideal partner.

That also falls into the realm of over pursuing or acting desperate, so you also need to remember communication is like a game of tennis; you don't hit twenty balls at someone, you hit one and wait for them to hit it back, so send one message and wait for a response. If you are sending way more messages to them then they are to you, then you come across as desperate and someone of not much value. Don't overwater a plant; it will die. You're better off to slightly under water than slightly over water.

Keep in mind that you are someone of value, so act like it. Your time is valuable; don't give someone heaps of your own time if they aren't willing to give you any, and make sure they are at least matching your input. That is what it really comes down to: input, and who is putting in the most. Hopefully, it is even; that should be the goal.

Where would you find your ideal partner? Well, remember on the list, you wrote down a bunch of hobbies you want them to have? Those hobbies are most likely similar to what you like, so if you love fishing, it would be great if your ideal partner also liked fishing or was at least open to it, so whatever your hobbies are, you should do them as much as possible because your ideal partner is probably doing the same. To summarise, with meeting them you should do the hobbies you love and be super friendly to everyone; I can't stress that enough. You need to be super friendly and chatty to everyone, so then if you meet someone else who is single, then you have a better chance of becoming a couple. If you are both single and doing a hobby you both like, but if either of you has a bad attitude, then there won't be any attraction; there will only be negative feelings.

If you want someone who is really positive, upbeat, and energetic but you are a cranky old fart, then they probably won't be attracted to you. That is where it falls into becoming what you want to attract again. Constantly work on this, always improving yourself, and building up more of your own potential. The more attractive qualities you have, the more appealing you will be to the opposite sex, and one of the most attractive qualities you can have is a great attitude, someone who is friendly, kind, positive, energetic, motivated, and ambitious. Easy to say but hard to come across.

I will lay out some simple steps on how to start to embody those traits. One of the biggest steps is surrounding yourself with people you want to become. Remember, you are a composite of the five main people you spend the most time with, so if your friends are fat losers who are negative all the time, then you will be on a fast track to embody the same characteristics. So slowly start transitioning your friends to people who are positive and motivated individuals. You may feel like you are dumping your old friends, but to clarify you do not have to straight out dump your friends, just limit the time you spend with them. So if you see one friend every day and they are a loser, start only seeing them once a week; just let the relationship fade away and grow apart. Find people who want to grow with you or are forcing you to grow faster; that is really the key to starting to improve your characteristics.

So you started hanging around winners who are motivated and positive, but what else can you do? Heaps actually. Start practising gratitude. Every morning sit down and close your eyes, think about three things for which you are truly grateful, and say thank you to the universe or to your god for giving you those moments or things. If you start every day saying thank you, then your life will change drastically for the good, and it will be a lot more positive after a few months. Science tells us that if you do something every day, then it will take 66 days to become a habit. This habit of saying thank you and priming your day for success is a perfect one to start today if you haven't already, and do it for at least 66 days. After that amount of time, if you haven't seen any difference, then try something else; how- ever, I am very confident this method will work great for you.

It is very hard to be a cranky old fart if all your friends are super positive winners and you do your priming and gratitude exercises every day, because these things will not only help you achieve a 10/10 relationship but also improve your life in many other ways as well. It is a really amazing thing I wish I did years ago. The human character is a very fragile thing; it can change so easily, but not always for the negative like you might be thinking; it can also change quickly for the positive, and it all starts with the beliefs we have. If you believe you are fat and ugly, then you will slowly morph into a fat and ugly person, so this means you need to change your beliefs.

The easiest way to do this is to change the script going on in our heads. During my priming exercise, I tell myself I am strong, I am incredible, and so on—all the things I need to hear to become the person I want to be. That is literally all you need to do to start to embody those traits. There's nothing magical about it; just change the script in your head.

At first when you start saying these super positive things to yourself, your brain will respond; it will respond with, "Bullshit! I am not strong. I am weak, I am a loser," but that is the old script fighting with the new one, and this is completely normal. However, it is important you don't let it win; just drown out that old script with the new one, saying, "I am strong, I am incredible," louder and louder, and over and over again until your brain believes it to be true, 110 percent. The brain cannot differentiate between what is real and what is imaginary. That is why humans are so affected by fear, whether it is based in reality or not.

Your own self-talk can truly make or break you. Don't underestimate it. Super successful people know they are champions, even before they become champions. Negative self-talk doesn't breed anything but more negativity. Some people believe you have to vent out any bad things that happen in your day—tell everyone about it until it is all talked out and vented. They think this will fix the problem or somehow ease the tension, but of course this is 100 percent false. Buddhists have known this to be untrue for thousands of years. Venting out your negativity doesn't fix anything or make you happier; it unfortunately has the opposite effect and makes you into a more negative person.

The only way to make yourself into a happier person and improve your perspective on any situation is to practice gratitude and make a plan on where to improve. If you complain about your job every day for 10 years, then that is your fault; instead, be grateful you have a job and an income and make a plan to start pursuing what you really want to do.

I used to be one of those people who would constantly complain about my job or the bad relationship I was in. I sounded like a little girl. (Quick tip here, guys: if you complain more than thirty seconds a day, then your girlfriend or wife will see you as feminine and her attraction for you will start to decrease, so keep that shit to yourself and practice gratitude and make a plan for improvement.)

Your ideal partner is a super, super important part of achieving a 10/10 relationship; it is impossible with the wrong person, so choose wisely, because you're going to spend the next fifty years with this person. Be super picky.

How can you increase your chances of finding your ideal partner? There was a great study done by Stanford University, showing the likelihood of meeting your ideal partner and where.

- At university/school – 9%
- At work – 11%
- At a club or bar – 23%
- Online – 40%

And the remaining percentage is made up from meeting your ideal partner through friends or family. So many people tell me all the time that they don't like online dating, or they have had a few bad experiences, but if you don't do online dating, you are literally cutting your chances down by 40 percent!

That's massive! If you haven't found your ideal partner and you really want to, you should definitely be using some dating apps or websites, because I predict this 40 percent likelihood will only increase in the years to come, so don't hold yourself back and convince yourself that you want to meet someone like your grandparents did. Times change, and you can meet your ideal partner anywhere, so increase your chances.

So some important takeaways from this chapter on finding your ideal partner:

- Write a super long, detailed list of exactly what you want.
- Be clear on what red flags you don't want to see.
- Become what you want to attract.
- Always be improving yourself.
- Leave the past in the past, and focus on the present and the future.

Dating

Dating is obviously an important part of relationships, since this is actually where most relationships end, before they really even start. That's the point. You are sorting through all the junk to find your ideal partner, your prince, your princess, etc. Hopefully, by this stage in the book, you have started on the journey to finding your ideal partner or you may have already found someone. Try not to worry; even if you have been married twenty years, this chapter will still provide you with a lot of valuable information because remember, the courtship never ends. You may have heard that many times but wondered what it truly means.

"The courtship never ends" means you must continually and forever be trying to increase your partner's attraction for you. I like to think of it like a fire, a campfire. If you just leave the fire and ignore it, it will eventually start to dwindle and slowly fizzle out. Relationships and attraction are the same; you need to constantly try to increase the size of the fire and increase the attraction. If you just ignore your relationship and assume everything will be fine and it will just be good forever, you are going to be sorely disappointed. The courtship never ends.

Personally, I like to take my girlfriend on a date at least once a fortnight, sometimes weekly, but usually every second week. I strongly recommend that if you're in a relationship, you go on a proper date twice a month.

You must be dating your partner forever. It never ends, so accept it and enjoy it. Some couples come to me asking for help, and one of the first questions I ask is, "When was the last time you two went on a date?" The answer is usually years, unfortunately. Nobody comes to me and says they go on a date every week, so never stop dating.

How we date is extremely important as well. Most people get this wrong and completely ruin the attraction-building. I'm going to tell you about the perfect date now. It doesn't matter how long you have been with this person, if it's the first date or the 1,000th one, do it this way every time.

Before I run you through the different parts of a perfect date, it is important to note that it is up to the man to date the woman, so guys this chapter is very important for you to study. As a man, you need to execute the date perfectly. The woman's job on the date is to relax and have fun; that is it, to be completely in her feminine energy and enjoy herself. The rest is up to the man.

The perfect date has at least a minimum of four parts:

1. THE PICK-UP

The pick-up/asking them out, is obviously the first step. Asking them out differs completely depending on what environment you ask them out at. If you meet on a dating site, online dating will be a lot different than meeting them at a club or somewhere in person, so one of the main things to remember is you must create rapport with this person. If you just walk straight up and say, "Would you like to go out with me tomorrow night?", you are going to get mostly no responses.

Creating rapport is a must. If you go up to someone and say "hello," then ask them their name, that's great, but don't offer up your name. This is a great test to see how high her attraction is to you. So if you say, "Hey, what's your name?" and she says, "I'm Sarah" in a low, monotone voice with not much eye contact, then the attraction is probably pretty low. If you say, "Hi, what's your name?" and she says, "HI! I'm Sarah. What's your name?" with a big smile and feminine voice, then her attraction for you is probably high. Understand the difference?

After this point, you just want to talk for a minute or two, then do the escape sentence: "Well, I'm going to see what my friends are up to. Can I have your number?" And if she gives you her number, do not ring or text her straight away! I have done this, and it is a massive attraction killer. You think, "Well, if I text her straightaway, then maybe she will want to hook up straight-away." Stupid idea. Take her number, give her a call in three to four days' time, and organise a date. Put the number in your phone and forget about it; then if you pass her again, just smile at her. If she wants to take it further or make a move, she will. If you chase her too much, she will start to lose attraction to you because you will come across as needy, desperate, or both.

Online dating is kind of the same, except the sentences are a bit different, but creating rapport first is still a must. Asking for their name is obviously stupid because you can already see it on their profile, so you need to come up with an opening line, something that makes them think, and which is an open-ended question. I used to use "If you could have any superpower, what would it be?"

I used to use that exact sentence, and it actually landed the beautiful woman I have in my life right now.

Think about these beautiful girls' profiles; they would have tonnes of men in their inbox constantly saying things like "Hey, how are you" or "Hey, how you doing?" Same shit over and over again, so you need to say something different and be creative. Ask a fun question like I did, really simple to start a good conversation, then after the conversation has been going well and rapport and attraction is building and it feels right, then ask her out on a date; it's really simple here, guys. Just say, "Would you like to go on a date with me this Friday night?"

It doesn't need to be complicated, and don't put too much pressure on yourself. Just ask the question really simply and fire it off. If you have built rapport and attraction properly, then she will say yes anyway.

Many people don't like online dating, because they think it's gross and everyone on there only wants sex. What I say to them is "Stop being so negative!" You must enter into this with an open mind. There are millions of people on online dating. Sure, some only want sex, but others want a proper relationship, and remember every good relationship starts as a casual fling anyway. People who skip the step of dating, or skip the dating period and pretty much just go straight into an exclusive relationship or even living together, straightaway are in for a very, very hard time.

2. THE ACTIVITY

The second step of the perfect date is doing an activity. Doing an activity sounds pretty dry and boring, but trust me, it is vitally important to a perfect date. When picking an activity, you need to pick something that is fun and physical.

My favourites are:

- Arcades
- Bowling
- Pool or snooker
- Mini Putt Putt
- Rock climbing
- Mountain climbing
- Walk on the beach
- Dancing
- Tango
- Club dancing
- Cooking together

All of these activities are physical. One of the worst activities you can pick is watching a movie, because sitting in the dark and staring in one direction for two hours is not a date. Now don't get me wrong, I love going to the cinema, but it does not count as a date, so get that out of your head right now.

Why does the activity need to be physical, you ask? Because it gives you the chance to be flirty, fun, and funny. It gives you a chance to grab her by the hips, use physical touch, and kiss. All these flirty, foreplay sorts of things will drastically increase the enjoyment of the date for both parties and increase the chance of sex at the end of the night as well as seeing that person again.

There is nothing worse than going on a date with someone you really like and then they never call you again. On the first date and every date for the rest of your life, you should be trying hard to raise their attraction for you. The higher you can get it, the better and more likely a 10/10 relationship will happen.

So, guys, always plan a really fun activity, *fun* as in what you want to do. Remember dates are always supposed to be secrets, so don't ask her what she wants to do, and don't plan the date around her likes. You decide what you want to happen, then execute in line with that. If you hate bowling but she loves it, don't go bowling. Make sure it's something you like as well. This is a great opportunity to make her laugh, be as funny as possible, be affectionate, and try to create the opportunity to kiss her.

3. THE MEAL

The third part of the perfect date is the meal, dinner. The majority of the time, guys, always plan for dinner dates/nighttime dates. Don't do lunch dates or breakfast, because day dates make it hard for sex to happen afterwards, so definitely try to only do nighttime dates, especially the first ten or so.

What type of restaurant you choose changes dramatically whether you're on your first date or one thousandth date. For a first date I always recommend a nice, medium-priced place. If you take a girl to a really expensive restaurant for a first date, it will come across as super desperate and needy, and she will feel that you are doing this to just get into her pants. So take it easy and find a nice medium-priced place. My favourite used to be a great burger joint with really top notch burgers, and dinner would cost about $70-$80.

Remember on a first date, the girl is just thinking, "I'm just going on this date to see what happens." She has no expectations, and she just wants to be super casual, so if you are thinking, "Damn, I really need to impress this girl, I better spend $500 on a meal," then there is a big disconnect there.

Communication is extremely important on the first date. Most people wreck it on the first date and never end up getting a second one. I want everyone to remember this simple rule: males only talk 30 percent of the time, females talk 70 percent of time. Guys, if you talk more than 30 percent of the time, then you will come across as a wanker. So ask the girl probing questions about herself, and keep her talking 70 percent of the time. If you do this, then her attraction for you will increase. Be mysterious and vague; this will also raise her attraction.

This is all about active listening. Active listening is a fantastic skill which will make you an all-around more attractive person, and it is the art of making someone feel heard. Sounds simple, right? Well it is, but the majority of people don't do it. The majority of people listen to someone talk and they already have a story lined up in their head, so regardless of what the person is saying, you already have a sentence you want to say about yourself. Most people are just waiting to respond instead of communicating effectively.

Probing questions is what you are going to use, so if she talks about her work, saying something negative about her boss or coworker, then ask a probing follow-up question like "Oh, why did they do that? or "Why did they say that?"

Probing questions will get the other person talking a lot more, they will feel heard, and let's be honest, people love talking about themselves. We have all spent time with that certain person who doesn't shut up about themselves, and they just keep talking and talking, and the entire time you're thinking, "Oh my God, I need to get out of here," while they are having the best time ever continually talking about themselves. So guys, regardless of how long you have been with your partner, whether it's a first date or you have been married twenty years, always practice the 70/30 rule for communication. I personally use it every day. Women love it, and so do my friends and family. Active listening is such a beautiful skill to use.

After you finish dinner, get up and go and pay, guys. I know society wants equality and to split the bill, but all this rubbish. Don't do that; you invited her on a date, so you pay.

Try to pick up on little hints. Is she leaning in towards you? Is she touching you? Is she looking at your lips? Try to see if she is giving any hints that she wants you to touch her or kiss her, and make your move at any stage of the date.

After you have finished dinner and are walking out of the restaurant, this is the time you want to go for a little walk and get the legs moving again. If you choose a place next to a river or beachfront or somewhere nice, then this can be a very roman- tic moment. This is also a chance to be a bit flirty, use physical touch, and kiss. You can ask leading questions, like "Do you know how to dance?" Then grab her and start doing the tango or something traditional but no twerking.

When you are dancing together and you can tell she likes you, look deep into her eyes, smile, then slowly lean in and kiss her.

After you have kissed her, pull away, take her by the hand, and keep walking and talking about something else, like it never happened. This will leave her a little confused but curious and aroused. Slowly walk back to the car and keep the conversation light, breezy, and fun.

4. THE DROP-OFF

During the drive home you should be keeping the conversation casual and using some humour to keep the mood fun. There are lots of ways to get her back to your house. For instance, you can use certain lines like "I have a beautiful dog at home. Would you like to see her?" Or "Hey, we should head back to my place and put on some music—it will be fun."

There are two different options there: the question and the suggestion. Both can work pretty well, or if you are a bit nervous and don't want to say too much, you can just drive to your house and then say to her "Come on" and wave her in, which works too. If she gives any kind of comment like "Not this time" or "No, I don't want to," then simply say, "Oh, okay, that's all right" and smile. Always smile. Then she will think in her mind, "Oh, he is really a nice guy," but if you get really emotional and seem really sad that she said no, then she will see you as weak and needy, which is very unattractive.

There are also some sentences or phrases you should never say at the end of a date. For example, never plan your next date on the one you're on, so never say, "This was great. Let's do it again next week."

That is a really dumb move because you are straight up destroying attraction and mystery. You need to keep her wondering, so don't say anything about how good the date was or any suck-up rubbish like that.

Some guys try to brown nose and really suck up to their date and go on and on about how pretty they are and how much fun they had. This is a bad idea. Keep your opinions to yourself, and always keep in mind that everything you do and everything you say affects your partner's level of attraction for you.

These rules always apply, guys, whether it's a first date or the 1,000th date. Never plan the next date on the date you are on! Be mysterious. She should be wondering how much fun you had, whether you are going to call her again, and if you like her. If she is wondering these things, then her attraction for you will increase.

After the first date, wait three to four days before contacting her, unless she contacts you first. These three days she will be wondering about you and hoping you will call, all while raising her attraction. She will be wondering what you're up to, what you think of her, and if you will see her again. This is exactly what you want, and it works extremely well.

Be aware if you are a "nice guy"; this may seem extremely difficult to do. If this is you, I recommend talking to four to five girls at once so you don't over-pursue any of them. Then, when you want to get serious with one, drop the rest. If you don't think this is you and can easily wait three to four days and let her chase you, then great.

If she sends you a message the next day saying how much fun

she had, then that is a great sign that she has high attraction for you. Don't ignore the message. Never ignore any messages, since a strong, confident alpha male leader never ignores people, even if they don't like them. Rather, they tell them how it is. However, if you are busy at work or whatever, take your time responding. You don't need to drop what you're doing to answer her like she's the Queen of England.

Stay in your masculine energy, guys. Girls, try to stay in your feminine energy. You may feel that it isn't very feminine to chase a man to get his attention and love, but it's actually extremely feminine, so don't feel ashamed to chase a man you like; it is a feminine trait.

However, there is a line of course, ladies. If you send him a message and he doesn't respond for seven days, then he has low attraction for you, and you should date someone else. On that note, girls, always use effective communication techniques. Remember, communication is like a game of tennis. Don't send him fifty messages in a row. Send one, then wait, and try not to send messages which are too long, because guys hate that. Keep it short or say it on a phone call. Personally, I haven't responded or even read some messages because they are simply too long. If you feel the message needs chapters in it, it is probably too long. When you go on a date with a man, stay in your feminine energy. Be affectionate, and push him to lead and make decisions. Be super joyous; it's very attractive.

And that is how you date properly for the best results. If you use all the information in the book, then you will become an expert at dating and relationships. Dating is often an overlooked part of relationships, and it is vital. The purpose of dating is to raise attraction. The more you increase attraction, the better the relationship will be and the longer it will last. Not only that, but dating is fun! So enjoy it and do it often; the more you do it, the better you will get. Practice!

Confidence

Confidence is extremely important in dating and relationships but also life in general. It is very difficult to achieve anything in life if you have low confidence. Say, if you're single and you see a really attractive person walking past, but unfortunately you have low confidence, so you don't say hello. You just let a great opportunity pass right through your fingers. Unfortunately, this is the case in so many scenarios, and people are their own worst enemy. I personally don't care how high your confidence level is right now, because it can always improve, and the higher it is, the more you will achieve, the better your life will become, and every single person around you will benefit as well.

Regardless of what stage of the relationship you are at (dating, exclusive, living together, engaged, or married), you need to be constantly working on your level of confidence. Attrac- tion and confidence are closely tied together. If someone is extremely pretty and has a great body but has low confidence, then your attraction for them will decrease like someone with a bad attitude. You don't want to spend much time with that person because it makes you feel down. If you start off dating someone and you are super positive all the time and have a high confidence level, then over time you start to become more and more negative and your confidence level goes down, your partner's attraction will definitely decrease with it. Be very aware of this.

As you can see, confidence is hugely important, and you should be constantly measuring your own confidence level. Ask yourself the question, "How confident do I feel today?"

To keep your confidence level high, there are a number of steps you can take:

1. SURROUND YOURSELF WITH THE RIGHT PEOPLE

First step is hanging around the right people. You have probably heard this again and again, and you may be sick of hearing it, but it is extremely important. Don't just hang out with anybody because you want friends; be picky. Ask yourself this question, "Will this person make my life better or worse?"

If they will make your life worse, then definitely don't spend time with them. Also, ask yourself that question with your existing friends. If you hang out with losers or people with low confidence, then you too will become a loser and have low confidence. You are merely a composite of the top five people you spend the most time with, so make those top five people the best fucking people you can find.

I love martial arts, so one of my top friends is a martial artist, another is a life coach, and another is a successful business- man. Your top five is crucial, and talking to them regularly is extremely important for becoming the person you want to be. So ask yourself these questions: "What sort of person do I want to be? What do I want to be good at?" This will give you the answer to what sort of friends you need to get.

Every time you spend time with someone who makes your life worse or brings you down, you are devaluing yourself. Do you want to be a champion and have a great life? Be picky with who your top five are. This can be particularly difficult for "nice people" because they don't want to stop hanging out with their loser friends, so if you don't want to dump them straight up, then do the "too busy" tactic, which is just making an excuse like you have work to do. It is basically lying, but it saves people's feelings (well, kind of).

Suddenly become "too busy" to hang out with certain people and spend all your time with winners, so every time they invite you somewhere or ask to hang out just reply that you have plans already or you are busy, and eventually the friendship will die. This may seem harsh, but the power of this first step is massive. If you want high confidence, if you want to be a champion, and if you want to achieve every goal you could possibly imagine, then you need to be very conscious of this rule.

2. PRACTICE, PRACTICE, PRACTICE

The second step in raising your confidence levels is practice, so if you want to get really good at talking to the opposite sex, then you need to practice.

Some of my clients, such as Jodie, who has low confidence and isn't a very good conversationalist, have set tasks to increase their skill set. For example, they must talk to at least five people of the opposite sex each week and try to make good conversation with them. The rule is they must be strangers, but if you do this enough times, your confidence will skyrocket. The first time you will be nervous, but the twentieth time you will be a natural; it just takes practice. Now Jodie is a fantastic conver- sationalist and extremely confident in herself.

Just like riding a bike, it takes time, and you are going to stumble and fall down a few times. You need to dust yourself off and jump back on, and before you know it you are a master. Every single thing in this book and in life works the same as that. Even though I laid out exactly how to execute the perfect date, the first time you try it probably won't be that good, but do it fifty times, and you will be a natural. Practice makes perfect, so if you're nervous or have low confidence, then just practice, talk to five different strangers and become a good conversationalist. If a super attractive person is walking past you, and you sound like Elmer Fudd, stuttering and sounding stupid, then there is a good chance that person is going to think you are disabled, and keep walking. So you need to practice.

Being a smooth talker is a very good skill, and girls, if you think you don't need to become a good conversationalist, then you are sorely mistaken. If you look great and you're nice, but you are terrible to have a conversation with, then high-value guys will give you one date and then never talk to you again. It is a massive turn-off, so practice and become charming.

3. TALK YOURSELF UP

The third step in raising your confidence is positive self-talk. The majority of people on this planet seem to talk very nega- tively about themselves all the time. They will call themselves stupid, fat, ugly, and all the negative things you can possibly imagine. If you have this kind of self-hating negative mindset, then why would anyone think any differently?

I have had dates with girls before who say, "If we sleep together tonight, then you won't ever talk to me again," and they say it so many times. One girl said it fifty times at least in one night, and she sold me on the idea, so I never talked to her again. If you are so negative and have low confidence and you communicate that fact, then whoever you are with will believe it, because you are selling them on the idea that you are a loser.

This is the exact opposite of what you should be doing. You need to sell them on the idea that you are a winner, that you are a champion, and if they don't talk to you again, then that is clearly their loss. Never, ever talk badly about yourself; be your own biggest fan.

I personally do this by morning priming, as I said earlier in this book. I wake up at 4:30 am every day (yes even Sunday), drive down to the beach, stand in the water, and do my prim- ing. I say to myself the things I need to hear to have super high confidence and be the man I need to be to achieve my goals. The sentences I say to myself over and over again while I stand in the cold water are: I am a strong, confident alpha male leader; I am strong; I am a champion; I am successful; I am a fucking beast; I will achieve everything I ever wanted; and I say them all with such conviction and certainty that the universe believes me.

If you say sentences like those to yourself every day for years, your brain will believe it! Remember what Tony Robbins' mentor Jim Rohn used to say, "You must stand guard at the door to your mind." That means whenever a negative or bad thought would come into your mind, you need to kick it out. Take that negative thought and fucking destroy it!

The words "I am a loser" never ever pop into my mind, and it even feels disgusting to write that sentence down. I know in my bones I am a champion, and there isn't a single thing that can convince me otherwise.

There will be tonnes of haters in your life; even your own family may discourage you. Many years ago when I became a relationship coach, everyone laughed at me, right in my fucking face. My "friends" at the time said I was stupid and begged me to stop because I was embarrassing them. I'm not going to lie; that hurt. Even my own girlfriend joined in on the laughter and mocked me.

You know who is laughing now? No one! Because I am successful, and I help people all over the world. People laugh at your dreams until they come true, then they say, "Wow, you're doing a great job," and I think, "Wow, not long ago you were mocking me," but I don't say it. I drop the resentment and just say, "Thank you," because being negative won't help anything.

This is a small taste of the haters in this world. Just be aware there are many people like this in the world, and the reason I didn't listen to those people even though it hurt a lot was because I knew in my bones that I am a relationship coach and my purpose on this planet is to help as many people as possible with relationships, so the opinions of others were never going to deter me from my purpose in life.

The track to success is hard and lonely. You lose more friends than you gain, but the friends you gain are of much higher value and much better people. I could've never achieved any of this if I didn't have high confidence, by continually telling myself over and over again what my purpose was and telling myself positive sentences every day that I needed to hear. I kept the confidence level high within myself so any hurdle which was placed in front of me, I easily jumped. A great sentence you can say to yourself is: I am strong, I am confident, I belong here, and people want me here.

4. SEEK EXTERNAL MOTIVATION

External motivation is motivation from videos, friends, or books. Believing in yourself is great, but others believing in you can make a big difference. I guarantee there will be times when members of your family say negative things about your goals or the method by which you want to achieve them. If so, you need to stand up for yourself—straight up! And say, "Hey! Don't you ever say that negative shit to me again! You want to keep talking to me, then keep those negative opinions to yourself!"

Sometimes you have to get mean, and you need to be upfront with people who don't support you. Every single one of your friends should support you. If you tell them your plans, they should say, "Oh man, that's great! Let me know if you need any help." Really nice and really supportive.

I hope this is starting to make sense. If you spend time with people who support you and motivate you to go harder, your confidence will be much higher, because it all compounds and keeps increasing. Negativity produces more negativity, and positivity produces more positivity; it's like a ball rolling down a hill—it gains momentum.

Another big external motivator is the content we consume: books, movies, TV shows, social media accounts, videos, and so on. Be very aware that the content you feed your brain affects it greatly. If you watch the news constantly, then it is going to be hard to stay positive, but if you watch motivational YouTube videos all the time, then you will probably be very positive.

It's the same with social media accounts. Go through your newsfeeds, and when you look at each account ask yourself the question, "Should I be consuming this person's content, or is it hurting me in the long run?" Very very few people ask themselves this question, but if you are on Facebook or Insta- gram for four hours a day, then that is a lot of content you are consuming. Best do a cleanup and make sure that content is positive and helps you to become the person you desire to be.

I personally think social media is fantastic, if it is used correctly of course. There is a lot of garbage and negativity on there, but that doesn't mean you have to consume that garbage or that gossip from your co-worker Karen. Unfollow! Unfollow! Unfol- low! Many of my extended family members have gotten upset because I have unfollowed them on social media. I do not care, because I only consume content that I want to consume and that will help me achieve my goals. Social media is a tool to be utilised, not merely enjoyed. Many Gen X people think social media is just for fun, but the younger generations know it's a tool to make money, build a business, or learn specific things.

So by the end of this chapter, I am hoping you have a few friends in mind that you don't want to hang out with anymore and that you are going to start practicing things to raise your confidence and you are starting to have an idea in your head about the type of friends you want. Hopefully, you have written down five sentences you are going to say to yourself every day so you can become the person you wish to be and, lastly, you have cleaned up your social media so you only consume what improves you.

Recap:

- Keep improving your top five friends.
- Practice, practice, practice.
- Do positive self-talk.
- Fill your world with positive external motivators.

PART IV

Communication

Communication

As we have talked about in previous chapters, communication is extremely important. However, it isn't the most important thing nor the least important thing, so relax.

Just kidding, don't relax yet; it is still very important! You will need to master this if you want to achieve a 10/10 relationship.

The way we communicate can make our partners like us or hate us; it can mean the difference between only getting one date or getting the person to fall in love with you. The most simple advice I can give on communication is to talk with your natu- ral energy. Men, talk in a masculine way, and females, talk in a feminine way. But what does that mean? Just the pitch? Men talk deep and women talk high? That does help, but it is a lot more complicated than that.

Girls, I bet you can remember a situation where you asked your partner to do something twenty times, and he still didn't do it, and you got more and more frustrated, and you asked the question, "Why don't you listen to me?" If you have ever done this, then it means you were not communicating effectively, so don't blame your partner. It takes two to tango, two to fight, and two to communicate.

Women that I coach like Michelle (and ones who want to be coached by me) often say that their husbands don't listen to them and they are bad communicators. After a few coaching sessions, the women see that their husbands aren't responding positively because of the way they are communicating with them.

Imagine it like this: If your partner speaks German and you talk to them in French, what do you think their response is going to be? They will be confused. Men often look at their wives with a befuddled look on their faces, thinking to themselves, "Why is she so angry?" So, girls, if you want your partners to listen to you and communicate better with you, then you must practice effective communication and communicate out of your feminine energy.

Communicating out of your feminine energy is so effective it's crazy! Girls, it works everywhere: with your partner, at work, with your kids, with your friends, everywhere! This is how you do it: Imagine you want your partner to take out the trash. You could say a masculine version, which would sound something like, "It would be *nice* if you took out the trash! I've only asked you ten times. You never listen to me."

How would he feel after hearing that? Would he feel good or bad? Quick tip everyone: If someone feels bad or criticised after you say something, then you were communicating ineffectively. If you communicate effectively, then the other person will feel good, maybe even motivated.

So you just saw how to communicate in a masculine way to your partner to take the trash out. On the other hand, a feminine way would be like this: you walk over to your man, slowly run your hands down his arms, slowly caressing him while looking up into his eyes, flutter your eyelashes and say in a sweet, feminine voice, "Honey can you please take the trash out for me?"

If you use this approach, you will find your relationship will improve dramatically. This is such an important tool to use, and it works extremely well. When you get really good at communicating from your feminine energy, then men will very rarely say no to you, and you can get pretty much anything you want.

Communicating out of your feminine energy also works well if you are at work. Even in a professional workplace, human nature cannot be ignored. Use this technique with whomever you are talking to. Obviously don't do the caressing part if it's inappropriate; however, you can still use physical touch in the workplace, even though technically it may be against the rules. Human beings love physical touch, so handshakes, high fives, a pat on the back, or a hand on the shoulder works great too.

Men, obviously that last section was just for the girls, but you should understand it too. You should be communicating out of your masculine energy, using decisiveness and leadership skills. This means remembering you are not a butler. You are the king of your castle! It is your role to lead your family to success.

The main thing to remember as a man is that women communicate mostly out of emotion and men communicate mostly out of logic, so sometimes a woman can say something which may seem quite mean. It may not be true; she is merely expressing how she feels at that moment. As an example, she might say, "You are a terrible partner!" You may have been a perfect partner for the last five years, but if you let her down today, she doesn't care that you were perfect for the first five years of the relationship. You fucked up today, and she is explaining how she feels out of emotion. This means to take what women say with a grain of salt, because it is not necessarily true or factual.

Guys, you might find times when your girl is upset and she doesn't want to talk about it, so what do you do? This particular technique took me a long time to learn, and I really struggled with it, and it can be very confusing for most guys. If your girl is upset and you can see it on her face that she isn't acting like herself, most guys ask, "What's wrong, baby?" And she simply replies with "Oh, nothing" and then the guy thinks to himself, "Oh, okay, I guess nothing is wrong. I'm going to go play Xbox."

Believe it or not, this is actually not the right approach to this situation. If you can tell she has something on her mind and she is being a bit moody or negative, you need to ask prob- ing questions in a nice way until it's resolved. Guys, females will test you with this, and it can get very frustrating. A few times with my girlfriend I would be probing her for an hour or more before she would tell me why she was upset. This can be very frustrating because it feels like you're getting nowhere. No matter how long it takes, you need to stay in the moment and keep probing her until you find out why she's upset. She will eventually tell you and air out all her feelings, and you will then be able to see that she is feeling better. The conversation doesn't stop until she is feeling better. This approach will make her really believe that you care about her feelings, but if you quit halfway through, then you are indirectly saying you don't care about her, which is not a smart thing to do if you want a 10/10 relationship.

So let's say you are probing her for a fair while and she eventually says that you hurt her feelings the other day with what you said, and it turns out you indirectly called her mother fat or something like that. Now remember, guys, women communicate out of emotion and men communicate out of logic, so she is going to tell you how that moment made her feel. She will say something along the lines of "When you said that stuff about my mum, it made me feel like you hate her and therefore hate me and it makes me feel like you don't care about me."

Now saying the words "I'm sorry" isn't necessary, and it wouldn't be effective anyway. You need to first build rapport by repeating half the sentence back to her. So you would say, "Oh, so when I said the comment about your mum, it made you feel really bad and somewhat unloved by me. That makes sense. I understand how you would feel like that."

By repeating back to her some of the words she has said, you are building rapport and saying "I understand" a lot; it makes her feel that you really understand and care about her feelings. You want to keep saying sentences like this until she has vented out all her bad feelings and there is room for positivity again.

The best time to handle a situation like the one we just went through is the exact time that it happened—not an hour later, not the next day, or next week; but as soon as you notice she seems a bit sad or a bit off, you need to handle it right then, ASAP. She may hit you with some objections, like "We need to go shopping" or "I need to make the bed" or whatever, but you need to stand your ground and say, "No, we aren't doing anything nor are we going anywhere until we have talked about this." Even if you have to physically stop her (in a nice way, obviously) from doing something else, then do so. The conversation must be had in the moment, ASAP. Remember, the purpose of this technique is not to make your partner think you are really sorry. The purpose is to make them believe you really care about their feelings and they feel heard and understood.

Here are some sentences you can say if she is refusing to talk about it:

- You don't want to talk about it?
- Remember a good relationship has good communication.
- Come on, tell me what's on your mind.
- Just give me a little hint.
- Tell me what's really on your mind.
- I really care about you, and I care about your feelings. Talk to me.
- You can talk to me about anything.

All these sentences work very well, and I use them a lot myself.

Society often tells us that honesty is the best policy. But is that necessarily true? It isn't true and here is why. It's safe to say if you are reading this book, you have some dating and relationship experience, and I'm sure at least once but probably more, your partner or the person you are dating has asked you how many people you have slept with or how many partners you have had. If we go by what society tells us, then we should tell them the truth, yes? If you have slept with fifty people, and then you tell them that, I can almost guarantee that their feelings will be hurt, regardless of whether they're a male or female.

Some questions you don't answer truthfully. If the answer is going to hurt their feelings and damage the relationship, then don't tell them about your past. The past is the past, and it doesn't matter anyway. The only thing that matters is the present and building a beautiful future, and that is exactly what you should tell them when they ask this style of question. So when my partner asks how many girls I have slept with, I respond "I'm actually a virgin." Now, this is funny because I have two kids already from a previous relationship, so it is obviously not true. If someone asks a bad question like this, respond with sarcasm, humour, or saying, "Look, baby, the past doesn't matter. I only care about the present and building a beautiful future with you." If you say that to someone, they can't help but agree with you and feel good about it.

And that all comes back to effective communication. When you say a sentence, how do you want your partner to feel? Your goal every time you communicate is to make your partner feel motivated, inspired, and positive; if they feel depressed, sad, or criticised, then it is ineffective communication. So every time, ask yourself, "How do I want my partner to feel?" This tech- nique is great not just in romantic relationships but also in work life, with your kids, coworkers, extended family, friends, every- one! Practice effective communication with everyone you meet all the time. Your life will improve dramatically, and the people you are communicating with will also feel happier, so just by communicating effectively you are making the world a better place. That's a huge difference compared to all these people yelling at each other and dishing out abuse, which is so sad.

If you handle any disagreements using effective communica- tion, they will not escalate into arguments. Remember, a 10/10 relationship has no arguments. If you two are arguing, then that means you both aren't using effective communication.

It can be very frustrating to act with lots of empathy and kind- ness when you are angry, so you need to take a breath, or even take a five-minute break if you have to, and then have the con- versation. You must make your partner and everyone around you believe that you do not tolerate arguments or drama in your relationship, and obviously you must believe it very strongly as well.

After any minor disagreement or situation where someone has gotten their feelings hurt, it is vitally important to do a twenty- second hug. I've done a few videos about this on my YouTube channel because it works so well. When you hug your partner, lots of feel-good hormones are released inside your body, and many of these are released around the twenty-second mark, so hold that embrace for at least twenty seconds and make it a nice big hug. Wrap your arms around tight and really try to feel the love. I honestly recommend that my coaching clients do this every day with their partners because it makes such a massive difference. People really underestimate how powerful some of these hormones are in the body, so use them to your advantage.

One thing all master communicators have in common is that they are very careful with the words they use. They realise some words carry a lot of weight behind them and can affect them personally. For example, there are many very successful business- men who refuse to use the word "tired," because they believe it to be defeatist and negative and it doesn't serve them in any way.

How often do you use language that is making your life worse? If you are reading this book, then you have probably had trou- bles with relationships in the past or maybe currently. Maybe the language you are using is negatively affecting you? At some stage you may have said, "All men are the same!" Or maybe, "All women are the same!" with negative connotations. This type of language isn't helping you; it's only making your present and future harder. Replace that bad language with positive things like "I love women, I think they're great" or "I think men are amazing." Just by speaking with more positivity, your brain will believe the things you are saying, and you will have much more luck in life. If you hear someone else speak with this kind of negativity, then pull them up and tell them to stop. Tell them you don't want to hear it. It will hopefully jolt them into rethinking their current style.

As you can see, communication plays a massive role in every-thing we do. If you pair effective communication with mastering masculine and feminine energy, then you will solve 99 percent of relationship problems. Unfortunately, mastering these things is actually quite difficult. I don't even consider myself a master at them yet, even though I do practice them every day.

You may have met someone one time in your life whom every-body liked. They had this power to make anyone smile, even though they were not attractive. What they did master was communication, and they had become an expert conversation-alist. You may be able to think of someone who makes you feel welcome, and they can make an amazing conversation with anyone. Try to learn as much as you can from these people. They have a beautiful skill and are often salesmen and people like that, or they may lie a lot, but you can't deny they are great conversationalists. It's a great skill. If you can master it, you will be able to strike up a great conversation with anyone you find attractive and get a great response.

As you are well aware by this stage, women test men all the time. I just helped one of my clients, Tim, who was having some trouble with his wife. They were running late, and she was still getting ready. He had all the kids ready to go, everything was ready, but everyone was waiting on her. He called me up and asked, "What should I do? She is getting angry and frustrated and isn't ready, and we are already fifteen minutes late." I replied with, "Just go."

It feels bad to do in the moment, but no one ever makes me late. Being on time is crucial, so I talked him through being emotionally stable and not getting sucked into the emotional fight she was trying to start, and she tried everything to get him to come back—loads of insults and low blows. I talked him through it, and he didn't get sucked into the fight. He stayed emotionally stable and after about thirty minutes, she had calmed down, and she hopped in the other car and went to where he was. When she got there, she said nothing.

He passed the test. She was angry and tested his strength and masculinity. He continued on with his day and communicated with emotional stability. The more he passes these tests, the fewer there will be; the more he fails these tests, the more times she will test, and each test will be harder. Guys, you have to pass every test!

Communication plays a massive role in everything we do. Most people take it for granted and don't think about it very much.

So an important takeaway from this book is to remember what effective communication is and learn how to use it to your advantage.

Advanced Communication

Advanced communication? Didn't we already talk about communication in the last chapter? We did; however, communication is so important that we are going to cover it again, but this time we are going to cover some advanced situations.

Guys, the first thing we are going to cover is the situation where your partner gives you the silent treatment because they are obviously upset about something. What should you do? At one stage or another, you and your partner will be upset with each other. Even if you are a master at relationships, enough years go by, and eventually you will be annoyed at each other because of something, so what should you do when she is giving you the silent treatment?

First step, realise that you will have no drama in your house, so if your wife starts bringing some drama in, you need to deal with it as soon as possible. Not the next day, not in a few hours, but right then and there. The moment you see she is upset or something is not quite right, you need to stop what you're doing and stop her as well and talk it out. Refuse to do anything or go anywhere until the situation is resolved. She will say things like "I have things to do," but you need to respond with "Too bad, nothing is getting done until we talk this out." Physically stop her in a playful way if you have to.

Then it is time to probe her. Most women when they're in this state won't surrender the information easily, so you have to probe them. You will have a long back and forth of you saying, "What's on your mind?" And she will reply with, "Nothing." This may happen over and over again, but eventually she will break and tell you what's on her mind and what has really been both- ering her. For example, she could say something along the lines of "It made me upset the other day when you said my mother was fat." The best response to this is "Oh, that makes sense. I can see how that would hurt your feelings. Me calling your mum fat was totally inappropriate and rude." At no point in that response did I beg for her forgiveness or say sorry, but I did make her feel like I care about her feelings.

The whole point of this is to make your partner feel like you really care about their feelings, that you understand their point of view, and you understand their pain. Being defensive or rude would do the opposite; that's why we never argue. If you replied with "I didn't say that!" Then your partner wouldn't feel like you care about her feelings at all. You must practice empathy in these situations and make her really believe you care about her feelings. This is the best way to handle any negative feelings or drama in your relationship.

Now your girl may be upset about something which has nothing to do with you; it might be about work or one of her hobbies. It doesn't really matter what the reason is. What is important is that you make her feel like you care about her feelings. This is quite a hard process and can be pretty stressful. You need to be patient with this, guys. Sometimes it only takes four minutes but other times it can take forty or more! Unfortunately, there is no shortcut. You need to take the time to clear the drama and let her vent her feelings. Once it is done, she will be saying things like "I feel better now" or "I'm glad we talked," etc.

If that's what guys do when a girl is upset, what do girls do when their man is upset? Guys, this is extremely important: a female can spend hours venting out her problems, but you can only spend five minutes a day. You may be thinking, "What? She gets hours to talk about her feelings, and I only get five min- utes? That's not fair!" Well too fucking bad! No one said life is fair. Men and women are different, so just accept it and accept human nature; don't fight it. The people who fight this end up in pain. You can't fight human nature. Guys, if you complain and whine about your day for more than five minutes, you are going to come across as a little bitch, and no one is going to find that attractive. Remember it's your job to be the leader. Your team will be reflecting whatever emotions you are showing. If you are being negative and weak, your family will show the same traits.

Girls, you may see your man is upset and he doesn't want to talk to you about it. Don't push him to talk or share his prob- lems. Him sharing his problems with his family won't make the situation better, only worse. If he must share them, then he can share them with me or a councillor or whatever—just not his wife and kids. So just leave him be, just concentrate on being feminine and positive, and be his joy.

Hopefully, it is clear now what to do when you sense drama in your home. Now another advanced communication technique is boundary setting. This technique or method can be used with anyone: your partner, kids, extended family, or friends. One of my clients, Sam, has trouble with his mother-in-law. (Actually, now that I think about it, almost all my clients have trouble with their mothers or mothers-in-law. Wow, I never realised that before, strange!) Well, anyway, I digress.

When setting a boundary, it is extremely important to do it quickly and aggressively. The slower and weaker you do it, the less chance it has of sticking, regardless of who you are setting the boundary with. I have coached my client Sam to be strong and direct with his mother-in-law. She often walked all over everybody and thought she was the boss everywhere she went and was not a particularly nice person. So now he has gotten to the stage of telling her exactly what he expects, and he pulls her up when she crosses the line. Most importantly out of all of this, his wife supports him. This is extremely important. If you are setting a boundary with someone and your partner is undermining you, then it will have little hope of sticking, unless of course you are a master at setting boundaries. This method requires a lot of self-discipline and strength.

I am very good at setting boundaries fast and aggressively. Even though I don't particularly like doing it, I would rather die than be a doormat and be disrespected. That is the mindset you need to have as well. Death before surrender. Like a Spartan soldier. Setting boundaries is important regardless of gender.

The first step in setting a boundary is you need to be super clear and super serious, because even the slightest vagueness or joking tone will undo you. The boundary needs to be very clear and simple to understand, so if a six-year-old can't understand it then it's too complicated. Some sentences which are good to say while setting a boundary are:

- Excuse me?!
- I will not tolerate that behaviour.
- Never ever speak to me like that again.
- Don't do that!

Eye contact is important with any of these. Aggressive eye contact and zero smile is a must to ensure they believe in every cell in their body that you are serious.

Very rarely does anyone disrespect me. I think people can just sense I will not tolerate it. One of my friends said to me, "If you give people respect, they will give it back." I replied with, "Bullshit!" He was quite surprised with my reply, and he said, "What?"

You see, you can be nice to someone and give them respect, and they can turn right around and be rude back. You can see this all the time in traffic and other situations. So how do people get respect? You have to give yourself respect first. If you give yourself respect and you have high value for yourself, then people will sense that and give you respect also. Or they could give you respect out of fear or intimidation. Personally, I don't really care as long as they are giving me the respect I deserve.

A few hundred years ago, if you disrespected someone, then you would have to duel them, and one of you would die, because they took respect seriously! Unfortunately, these days most people are doormats and get disrespected constantly and do nothing about it. I see this constantly in relationships, with a couple, for example, that has been married for decades, and the wife treats her husband like shit, like he's her slave. She'll say, "Do this, do that," and all he replies with is "Yes, dear." Pathetic!

Guys, even though some women think they want this, trust me no woman actually wants this! Every single woman alive wants to be with a strong, confident alpha male leader; that's why it's fine to do things for your wife but tell her no sometimes too. You are not her slave, and it is not your job to make her happy. In fact, the more you do for her, the worse you are making her life. She is becoming reliant and weak and stepping into her masculine energy which she really doesn't want to do.

I constantly hear guys saying, "Oh I just want to keep the peace" or "Oh, it's not worth the fight." Are you fucking serious!? It is always worth the fight, every single time! Guys, you need to have the mindset like a Spartan warrior, never surrender. You win or you die trying. "It's not worth the fight" is such a feminine, weak thing to say. Are you a doormat or a man? Are you weak or strong?

Guys, if you display this level of strength and confidence, your wife won't argue with you anyway because she will see you as too strong and realise it is not worth the battle. If she disagrees with you or is upset, she will bring it up in a nice, controlled, mature way. Never accept anything less. Never accept any level of disrespect from anyone.

Girls, I understand this would be easy if your man was a strong confident alpha male leader. It is very hard if he is not, but be aware that how you treat your man will either make him more masculine or less. If you are really bitchy and mean to him, he will naturally become more feminine unless he has learnt how not to. If you are nice, feminine, and girly, he will naturally become more masculine. You need to force him to lead; nobody becomes masculine by accident. People become masculine out of necessity. You need to make it a necessity for him. Give him all the responsibilities, all the hard stuff, all the decisions, and let him handle it. Life will make him more masculine. Then you stand by his decisions and enjoy the journey. By being really mean and bitchy, you will not make your man more masculine; it will make him more feminine, unfortunately.

As you can see, communication is so important, and how we communicate and what we tolerate is important. In fact, communication is so important that if you get into a relationship with someone who is a bad communicator, the chances of the relationship ending go up dramatically. Therefore, you need to learn how effective communication and advanced communication techniques work.

Becoming a good conversationalist—what does that mean? Think back. Have you ever known anyone who could make a conversation with anyone and it was a good, positive conversation? Usually people like this are pretty hopeless at everything else. They are usually overweight and not very good-looking, so they pretty much have nothing going for them, but they are fantastic conversationalists, and they have the gift of gab. Becoming a good conversationalist is such a valuable skill that it will help you immensely with relationships, getting jobs, raising kids, everything.

But how do we learn this skill? Practice, practice, and more practice. Just like everything in life, you need to practice it to be good at it. Join ten different social clubs; this will force you to have tonnes of conversations with all sorts of random people. Have random conversations with random people. Become a salesman. Salesmen are usually pretty good conversationalists because they rely on it to make money. Study the Wolf of Wall Street, Jordan Belfort, who wrote a book about selling. A lot of the book is about building rapport and how to get people to like you. Another great book to read about this is *How to Win Friends and Influence People*, an amazing book written during the great depression I believe. I've read it about fifty times. Both of these books show you how to become a good conversation- alist and show you how to get people to like you.

A quick tip is to talk about them and get them talking about themselves. The conversation should focus on the person you are talking to, and rarely talk about yourself. A quick way for people not to like you is to constantly talk about yourself. If you know anyone who is a good conversationalist, then study them and learn their technique.

Someone who has the gift of gab has a way of making you think you want them as your best friend, that they are always there for you. They make you feel emotionally safe, and you look up to them at the same time. Do you make anyone feel emotionally safe? It is a very powerful trait and one you should practice.

There are so many potential situations I could cover under advanced communication. One I want to cover is when you should tell a girl you love her or propose? This is a really simple one. A girl will drop little hints when she wants you to propose. She will be looking at rings or looking at wedding stuff. If she isn't doing any of that or saying anything related to that, then she isn't ready yet. Similarly, with saying "I love you," after you are dating someone for two to three months, you should see it in their eyes, and you should almost be able to feel it, until you can't hold it back anymore and both of you want to say it.

Don't rush these things, guys. The universe will tell you when the time is right, and she will tell you too. You will see all the signs. Many guys propose too early because they are deeply in love, but the girl isn't ready to be engaged. She just says yes because she doesn't want to hurt your feelings, so just wait until she is dropping heaps of hints. Girls drop a lot of hints about a lot of stuff; you just need to be listening and watching her to pick them up.

I personally hate hearing the sentence "My partner is so hard to buy for." In relation to presents, if your partner is hard to buy for, it means you aren't paying attention and you're a bad partner. You should know your partner so well that you know exactly what types of things they like and what will make them feel the most loved. If you ever say that kind of negative sentence, strike it from your vocabulary because it's not helping you; it's hurting you. Your partner is easy to buy for. Just listen to them.

It really amazes me how defensive people are. I guess it comes from their ego. When I do a group call with a couple, I do a little technique where each person gets to choose one thing their partner has to do. So say, for example, the husband might say, "I want her to spend an hour with me before bed just talking and stuff." Easy, right? Then the wife usually says something that is far too vague and confusing.

Quick side note girls: Men's brains don't comprehend information like yours does. Men need super clear, simple instructions. Women will often say things like "If you see something needs to be done around the house, then just do it without me having to ask." Now, this is a super terrible sentence because it's opinion based. He might think the house looks amazing, and she may think it looks terrible, so it's up for debate. Instead, when communicating with someone, try to avoid this mistake and make your instructions super clear and non-opinion based.

So back to the couple on the group call. The man would ask for an hour of her attention before bed, in which most women get immediately defensive and say things like "I do spend time with you before bed!" Or "You are busy on your phone anyway, so why does it matter?" Super terrible way to communicate, girls, and it's super mean. If you are being defensive, then you are not communicating effectively. Remember that!

Of course on the group call when the wife acts like this, I put a stop to it immediately and lecture them on effective communication. Many, many women say their husbands are bad communicators, but over my years of coaching, I have actually found that women are worse at communicating, much to my surprise. So, girls, if you are reading this, take it upon yourself to break the cycle of bad communication, and become an effective communicator. The woman's request is usually something along the lines of "Every morning can you make the bed." The husbands in my experience always say, "Yep, easy," and husbands seem to rarely get defensive in this exercise which is great to see.

After this exercise is over, both people have learnt a lot about communication, which is amazing. Then I make them face each other, look each other in the eyes, and say three things they like about each other's bodies. Everyone is always surprised by this, and it's very funny. I find most people aren't totally happy with their body, so it gives them a boost and makes them feel attractive. Then after they each say three things and have a laugh, it's time for a twenty-second hug. And that's the end of the call.

In conclusion, these advanced communication techniques are super valuable and important. Learn them and, more importantly, put them into action today!

PART V

Intimacy

Sex

When we talk about intimacy, the fifth and final pillar of any successful relationship, we must of course talk about sex.

Without a 10/10 sex life, you do not have a 10/10 relationship. Many couples struggle in this department; everything is a 10/10, except the sex, and they have trouble raising it above an 8/10. So what can you do?

Believe it or not, everything I cover in this book has to do with sex in one way or another, so if you implement everything you read, your sex life will improve—such as utilising the love language theory created by Dr. Gary Chapman. If you com- municate your partner's love language, then everything will improve. If I could sum it up in a short description, everyone has specific ways they feel love the most, and there are five categories. They are:

1. Words of Affirmation
2. Physical Touch
3. Gifts
4. Acts of Service
5. Quality Time

Which two of these do you enjoy the most? Then out of those top two, which one could you live without? And there you have it, that is your love language. If you know your partner's love language, it will improve your relationship.

Along with love language, you also need to master masculine and feminine energy, since this plays a massive role in sex and attraction. Guys, if you are more masculine, your woman is going to be more attracted to you, which in turn will increase sex frequency. The lower her attraction is, the less she will feel like it. We must raise that attraction as high as possible. Communication also plays a massive role. If you are a terrible communicator and haven't mastered effective communica- tion yet, then that will also impact your sex life. As you can see, everything affects it in one way or another. Just remember though, the higher the attraction, the more frequent and better the sex is.

One of my favourite lines from my old coach was "Sex must be the man's fault." I spent years pondering over that sentence. I was very confused and wasn't really sure what it meant. I thought to myself, *I've had heaps of great sexual experiences where she initiated it*. But technically if she starts things off and leads the entire experience, she is in her masculine. Girls like to be chased, they like to be hunted. Even when I know my part- ner wants to have sex like crazy and needs an orgasm, she still likes to put up a bit of a fight and say, "No, it's okay, it doesn't matter." Then I grab her and throw her on the bed and pull off her clothes, and the biggest smile appears on her face, and on occasion she even starts singing out of joy when the act begins.

I now fully understand what my coach meant when he said sex

must be the man's fault. By being in my masculine and taking control of the situation, and seducing her and giving her the opportunity to put up a fight, it allows her to stay in her feminine, which is what she wants and what she needs. She wants sex to be my fault. Girls don't want to be in their masculine and be responsible for the sex. They want to be chased, hunted, and seduced.

Through all of my learning about relationships, it makes me reflect on my previous relationships, and it makes me just shake my head. I did so many things wrong! I fucked up every day. I'm just glad I know now. Some people I coach are in their 50s and 60s, and they are still having trouble. But I guess it's never too late to learn.

The other part you need to learn about having an amazing sex life is the erotic blueprint. The erotic blueprint concept was created by sexologist Jaiya, and she has made a free test avail- able online to help you identify your type. Learning about what blueprint you are and what your partner is will improve your sex life a lot. It has improved mine quite a bit. I have learnt a lot about myself that I would have never known if I had never done the test.

Understanding each Erotic Blueprint Type is like getting the secret decoder ring to becoming a sex-life superhero and claiming your own satisfaction and fulfilment. Here is a quick look at the five Erotic Blueprint Types.

EROTIC BLUEPRINT #1: ENERGETIC

Aroused by space, anticipation, and teasing. They are very sensitive and need time to assimilate to sexual touch; too much too fast turns them off. If you enjoy a lot of foreplay and like to experiment with different toys, massage oils, and other props, you probably have this blueprint.

EROTIC BLUEPRINT #2: SENSUAL

Aroused by sensation: touch, sound, taste, smell, etc. They bring beauty, comfort, and whole-body sensuality to a sexual encounter. Their biggest turn-off is being stuck in their head and living in tension. A Sensual Type needs to be relaxed to open to sexual connection and turn-ons. If you need to create the right environment to be turned on and get excited when the right lighting, music, and smells are present, this might be your blueprint.

EROTIC BLUEPRINT #3: SEXUAL

Aroused by the simple act of intercourse. Sex is fun, and they use sex to relax. Those with this sexual style are ready to get down to business whenever there's time or a willing partner. However, they can get stuck in a limited view of sexuality and can be goal-oriented.

EROTIC BLUEPRINT #4: KINKY

This type is aroused by the taboo. But they oftentimes have deep shame about their taboo desires and, if they don't have a supportive partner who deeply listens to their needs, they can suppress their type and become distant or develop self-esteem issues.

EROTIC BLUEPRINT #5: SHAPESHIFTER

Aroused by all of the above. They are endlessly creative but need a partner who is also equally adventurous. Sometimes they shift to be what others want them to be instead of owning their own sexuality, needs, and desires. Shapeshifter types often have to take time to reconnect with themselves so they can be more authentic and vocal in their sexual preferences.

As Tony Robbins says, the first step to transformation is to "take massive action," so go out there, get some great mentorship, get fully authentic with yourself and your partner, and learn how to speak each other's erotic blueprints! That's the path to more erotic pleasure, more desire, and more intimacy in your relationship.

My erotic blueprint test results show that I am half Kinky and half Sensual. Some of the sensual things I like are slow dancing with my partner while listening to romantic music and staring into each other's eyes, which makes me feel very loved and surprisingly horny. I always wondered why I like that so much. The kinky side of my personality likes things that other people may find weird or wrong like rim jobs and spitting. These things I find extremely satisfying and quite the turn-on. Having an understanding and open-minded partner is extremely import- ant here, because if you want your partner to spit on you and you ask, but your partner responds with judgment and disgust, then you will feel adrift and that would be very sad. So it is very important to go into this with a very open mind and an open heart.

In saying that, though, you don't need to do everything your partner desires. If your partner likes a certain thing, but it is just too much for you, then it's okay to say, "Hey, I totally understand you like that, but I just can't at this stage—it's just too much for me at the moment." They should understand. For example, if your partner really wants to watch porn with you, but it is just a massive turn-off, then it's okay to say no, or find a happy medium somewhere. What is good about the erotic blueprint is that you get a really good understanding about who your partner is, who you are, and how to please yourself and how to please your partner. If your partner wants to watch porn with you, but you really really don't want to because you are self-conscious about yourself, then a happy medium could be a movie with soft-core sex in it, or certain types of porn that don't make you feel bad, like a cartoon or something. So there is always a happy medium somewhere.

One thing to remember is that your results can change and adapt over the years, so it's a fluid process. Be open to change and enjoy it.

Something that makes me very sad is when I'm coaching a couple and the woman says, "After a long day at work the last thing I want to do is have sex." That is a very sad statement. Since when did your job become more important than your relationship? Girls, if you take sex out of a relationship, the feelings of love and positivity your husband has for you will quickly turn into angst and hatred. I can't be more blunt about this: taking away love, affection, and intimacy is a superfast way to get to a divorce. So for fuck's sake, sleep with your husband! He must feel satisfied and happy with your sex life or trouble will arise, regardless of how perfect you are in every other area. I have seen so many relationships end because of a bad sex life. Don't be one of them!

Often women complain to me about their husbands, telling me that their husband complains a lot or seems stressed or insecure. Guess what the answer is to these problems? Affec- tion! Insecurities can be silenced with more affection. If your partner has some insecurities about you being friends with the opposite sex, for example, all they are really saying is that they aren't getting enough love and they feel like some of your love is going to someone else. If they feel 110 percent satisfied and happy in every department, then they aren't feeling cheated and they won't feel like they are missing out, so understand your partner's insecurities for what they really are: a hidden message telling you they need more quality time and affection.

If a couple has sex every single day and has a 10/10 sex life, they will rate the relationship higher as well. Your sex life affects your relationship massively, so don't take it for granted and don't say sentences like "Men only care about sex." Who cares if this is true or not? If you don't like men, go out with a woman. That's how men are. Don't try to change them. Accept them for what they are. And men, never say the sentence "All women are the same, they are all a pain in the ass." These kinds of terrible, neg- ative sentences will only hurt your future and hurt the chances of you ever achieving a 10/10 relationship.

Jim Rohn said, "Stand guard at the door to your mind," and it is so true. Don't let yourself have negative thoughts. We all have negative thoughts sometimes, but what I like to do when I have a negative thought is to reach inside my head, grab the thought, and crumple it up like a piece of paper and throw it into the bin. When I have a negative thought about my partner, I stop myself as soon as possible and I say, "No! She is not like that, she is a great person and she is lovely and I love her deeply," or something along those lines. Controlling your thoughts and your words radically changes your life in so many ways, so if you don't do this at the moment, definitely start doing it, and eventually you will master it. It is very hard to have a 10/10 relationship when you have non-stop negative thoughts about your partner. I would say it's impossible to be successful at anything in life if you have negative thoughts about that thing all the time, so stand guard at the door to your mind.

A few other things to remember about sex: it isn't your job to make your partner happy, so put yourself first. Many people struggle with this, and they will put their partner's needs first, but then no one ends up having a good time. There is nothing worse than when you're having sex with someone and they are pulling a face which makes you think they aren't enjoying it; that's such a massive turn-off. It is very hard to hide discomfort, so if you aren't having fun, no one is. So use effective commu- nication and tell your partner what you like and ask them what they like. You are going to spend many, many years with this person, so the sex should be fantastic. Put all these techniques into place and you should have a 10/10 sex life.

The one thing we haven't covered is your physical state. If you are severely overweight, have hormone issues, or are just gener- ally really unhealthy, then you are going to have trouble sexually. This is a big one for guys, because there is nothing worse than a limp dick when it's time to perform—it's super embarrassing and you feel like a real loser. So guys, if you sometimes have this issue, then it could be a number of things. First, it could be performance anxiety, which means you are simply just thinking about it too much. You may be saying to yourself, "Stay hard, stay hard," but then it goes soft. Not great!

or something along those lines. Controlling your thoughts and your words radically changes your life in so many ways, so if you don't do this at the moment, definitely start doing it, and eventually you will master it. It is very hard to have a 10/10 relationship when you have non-stop negative thoughts about your partner. I would say it's impossible to be successful at anything in life if you have negative thoughts about that thing all the time, so stand guard at the door to your mind.

A few other things to remember about sex: it isn't your job to make your partner happy, so put yourself first. Many people struggle with this, and they will put their partner's needs first, but then no one ends up having a good time. There is nothing worse than when you're having sex with someone and they are pulling a face which makes you think they aren't enjoying it; that's such a massive turn-off. It is very hard to hide discomfort, so if you aren't having fun, no one is. So use effective commu- nication and tell your partner what you like and ask them what they like. You are going to spend many, many years with this person, so the sex should be fantastic. Put all these techniques into place and you should have a 10/10 sex life.

The one thing we haven't covered is your physical state. If you are severely overweight, have hormone issues, or are just gener- ally really unhealthy, then you are going to have trouble sexually. This is a big one for guys, because there is nothing worse than a limp dick when it's time to perform—it's super embarrassing and you feel like a real loser. So guys, if you sometimes have this issue, then it could be a number of things. First, it could be performance anxiety, which means you are simply just thinking about it too much. You may be saying to yourself, "Stay hard, stay hard," but then it goes soft. Not great!

10/10 sex life is super important, and your relationship isn't a 10/10 unless you have a 10/10 sex life. Get it to a 10/10. I know you can!

Growing Together

I have taken many phone calls over the years from couples, and they say the age-old sentence, "We are drifting apart."

But why? Why do people drift apart?

Quick question: Are you still friends with your first best friend? From school? I know I'm not, but why not? We used to do everything together. We loved sport and we would play it three times a day and we were so passionate about it. We were unbreakable, but then over the years we slowly drifted apart. I left school and started my apprenticeship, and we hardly talked, and I didn't see him again for about four years. We were both adults then, standing there, staring at each other with nothing to say, with nothing in common, both thinking to ourselves, "Boy, this is weird!"

Human beings seem to have quite a short memory. We can be inseparable one minute and complete strangers the next, and years and years go by, and you have no desire to reach out to them, even though you probably could if you really wanted to. It's sad when you start to think about it.

My educated guess on why human beings do this goes back to when humans lived in small tribes up to 150 people, thousands of years ago. If you only knew 150 people, it wouldn't take long until you knew everyone well, and you wanted to breed to have offspring, but if you group up there, then it could be damaging for the tribe because of incest and other problems that arise in that department, so they would leave the tribe to find a new tribe and breed with those people. Thousands of years later, we have gone from ten thousand people on the earth to billions, so this is a very effective method.

Our brains and emotions also let us and want us to do this. If we were super strongly emotionally tied to our families so we could never leave, then the human race would die out and go extinct, so the feeling of wanting to leave your family as soon as possible when you're almost an adult is an important one and essential for breeding strong human beings. This is also very easy to see in the animal kingdom—all male animals when they get to a certain age either challenge the leader or leave to find another pack, and humans aren't much different. That is my educated guess on how it's so easy to drift apart from someone to whom you were once so close.

So what does all this history stuff have to do with relationships? A lot, actually. To understand our pasts and to understand our nature helps us better understand ourselves and why we do certain things. That is why I'm never surprised when a couple starts drifting apart. It is natural.

So you may be asking yourself, "Is it even possible for a couple not to drift apart or are we all doomed?" It is possible, and I'll tell you how; it's called growing together, and it has several steps.

1. COMMON GOALS

If two people are constantly working on a common goal or against a common enemy, then they will have something to bond over. Remember, opposites attract, but similarities are what bond us. If you are both working together every day on a common goal, it is very hard to drift apart. That commonal- ity is why you see so many successful entrepreneurial couples working together on their business and they seem so happy. I'm sure they have some disagreements, but overall they are working together towards a common goal.

Many very successful billionaires have their wives helping them along every step of the way. I believe it is actually impossible to become successful without the support of your partner. So find a common goal, whether it is business, kids, sport, or whatever. The goal doesn't really matter as long as you are working as a team to achieve it.

2. DUAL HOBBIES

This one is really all about spending quality time with your part- ner doing things you both enjoy or are open to. My partner and I have lots of different hobbies, so once a month or fortnight we will do something that we don't normally do, like play squash or golf. Those activities are a great bonding exercise and always bring us closer together, and it's a lot of fun.

It doesn't necessarily have to be something you both love. For instance, I love Karate, but I don't expect my partner to join me in that. Rather, we do abstract things we wouldn't normally do, like golf. We may play golf once a year, and we are terrible at it, but it's a lot of laughs, and we can have a few drinks, play some music, and just have fun. Neither of us particularly enjoys golf, but that doesn't matter—it's just for fun. Now if you really think about it, I'm sure you can think of at least ten things you would only do once a year. Guys, here is a little tip for you: the more you can push a girl out of her comfort zone, the higher her attraction will be for you, so pick things that make her heart beat fast, push her to the limits, and lead her through it.

3. HAVING A 10/10 RELATIONSHIP

This one is kind of self-explanatory, but I'll explain it anyway. If you follow everything in this book and get your relationship to a 10/10, then you are far less likely to drift apart, because people who hate each other drift apart much faster. If you have a 10/10 sex life, then you are less likely to drift apart; if you go on holidays all the time, then you are less likely to drift apart; if you are both effective communicators, then you are less likely to drift apart; and if you both know how to keep your partner's attraction at a 10/10 then, you are less likely to drift apart.

There you have it—three basic steps everyone can follow and understand. If you follow all these things, hopefully I won't be getting an email from you saying "My husband and I have been married fifteen years, and we just seem to have drifted apart, the spark is gone, and we don't really enjoy spending time together." I've built a business out of helping people with relationships, but hopefully, for your sake, you'll help yourself with this book before it gets to that stage.

Most people I coach come to me when they are in massive pain, and I say to myself, "I wish they would have come to me six months earlier, because it would've been so much easier."

However, that's not how humans work. They are only ready for change when their pain threshold has been met. It's sad, really. Most people put up with what I call "mild discomfort." For example, they say their job is okay, they say their relationship is okay, they have a mild discomfort with it all but not enough pain to do anything about it. I used to fit into that category as well. I was in emotional pain for years, but it was never bad enough for me to really change.

I don't wait for pain anymore. Now I'm always striving for better, I'm always striving for success. I used to be reactive, but now I'm proactive. "Good things come to those who wait?" What a load of bullshit! Success doesn't come to those who wait. Success comes to those who are hungry enough to take massive action consistently so the universe has no choice but to hand over success to them. I could easily be sitting on the couch watch- ing TV right now, but instead I'm sitting in my office writing this book. I don't wait for anything. I go get it! "Be aggressively patient." I love that sentence. "...aggressively patient." Really think about that.

Sometimes two people are just so different that they will never get along. It has been many years since I broke things off with my ex, and we still don't get along. We never did, and regard- less of how much I try, it seems we never will, but that's okay because you aren't going to get along with everyone you meet. You can't make everybody happy, but you can make yourself happy. If you are in a relationship that is so dreadfully bad that no matter what happens you just can't see it improving, and no matter what happens you don't think you will ever get along with your partner on any level, then it's time to leave. Unfor- tunately, you aren't compatible. Unless both of you are really open to being coached and really open to hard change, then just end it and find someone more compatible with you. There are billions of people on this planet, so don't get hung up on just one.

As human beings I think we find it difficult to end a relationship with someone because of our egos. We don't want to be seen as quitters. We don't want to be seen as weak or bad people so we stick it out. We hope that tomorrow will be a better day regardless of the fact that the relationship has been bad for years. There are a lot of hard truths in this book which will make you ask yourself some big questions in life. I know it's difficult, but you are the architect of your own life, so you need to ask yourself these big questions.

Let's talk about TV. The conversation about TV comes up a lot. Many people say, "My partner doesn't want to watch what I want" and vice versa, and it always makes me laugh. Take a step back and breathe for a second and remember it's just TV. TV preferences don't matter, because what is more important is that you are together.

One couple I coached a while ago, Eli and Shaun, were struggling in their relationship. She liked to watch *The Bachelor* and he hated it, so they would watch TV in different rooms. What is the solution here? There are so many different options on what you could possibly do. In their situation, the best solution was for her to download all the episodes and watch them at a better time and to have sex with each other instead. You may be thinking, "Wow I didn't see that coming!" Sex was an issue for this pair. They mastered everything but struggled in the sex department, but eventually we got that to a 10/10 too. She was stuck in a loop of saying "no" and felt she should only do it when she felt like it, but she learnt very quickly that if you starve someone of affection and intimacy, then the love and positive feelings they have for you quickly turn into hatred and angst. I have seen so many relationships end because the sex life was bad. Just do it!

Letting something so silly like TV affect your relationship is madness and that goes for social media as well. Some people are quite content to sit on social media all day, scrolling through their feed, looking at stupid shit and ignoring their partner. Here's the thing to remember: If you ignore social media, it will still be there when you get back. If you ignore your part- ner after a long enough time, they won't come back. So turn off the TV, turn off your phone, and spend some quality time with your partner. Time is so precious and life is so short, so use your time wisely now before it's too late. You can't get time back once it's gone.

If you don't consciously grow together, you are doomed to drift apart. Heed this warning and use the advice in this book. I believe the greatest tragedy in life is to absorb knowledge but never put it into action. Don't let this be you! Use the knowledge, put it into action, and become a winner.

Relationship Timeline

Most people move too fast in relationships. I have in the past as well. You meet someone you are somewhat attracted to, then within one month you are basically living together and pregnant.

Not following the relationship timeline is like building a house on the mud without foundations; it will eventually fall over. It takes time to build foundations. The foundations in relationships are things like trust, characteristics, and just getting to know each other. It takes time, so in this chapter I'll explain the best time to do certain things in a relationship for the best results.

0-3 MONTHS

This time is just for dating. You are not exclusive. You are just spending some time with each other, going on dates and having a good time, with no pressure and no worries. This time is really for building up the foundations, learning as much as you can about that person, and slowly building that trust and attraction.

In these first three months, you should be watching their actions when you are with them and asking yourself the question, "Is this something my ideal partner would do?" For example, if the person you are on a date with pulls out some hair from his or her pocket and puts it in the meal in an attempt to get a free meal, you should ask yourself, "Is this something my ideal partner would do?" And if the answer is "no" too many times in a row, then they aren't your ideal partner.

Personally I recommend talking to four to five different people at this stage of the dating process. If you are really serious about finding your ideal partner, you need to increase your odds a little bit. You don't need to sleep with all of them—just talk and get to know them, and if that person isn't your ideal part- ner, then rotate them out for someone new and keep going and dating people until your ideal partner comes into your life. Most people completely skip this stage and go right into being exclusive, and they know nothing about one another and are in for a world of hurt. So slow down, go on a date once a week, and get to know each other. Then, after two to three months, you should both want to say, "I love you"—that's when it's time to go exclusive, or make it "Facebook official."

3-9 MONTHS

This period you are dating exclusively and not talking to any other potential partners. If you are still talking to other people, then stop! You are not being congruent with your goal of getting your relationship to a 10/10. Be with the person you are with 110 percent or not at all.

During this period of dating, you are really starting to fall deeply in love with each other and starting to make plans together for the future. This is not the stage to move in together. Even if you spend every night in the same bed, you are not technically living together yet; that is the next stage. All you do in this stage is spend lots of time together, meet each other's fami- lies and friends, have a good time, and slowly start to plan a bright future together. This is also a very good time to set strong boundaries so your partner knows what you like and tolerate and what you don't like and refuse to tolerate. By the end of this stage, you should both trust each other 100 percent and should be honest with each other.

I think people, including myself, have skipped over these stages in the past because emotions get in the way, and emotions want you to do things superfast. As animals, we want to find a partner and get them pregnant the same day, but that is not an effective strategy if we want to be with this person forever.

9-12 MONTHS

Now this is the time when you both get serious about moving in together. Before nine months, it is too early, so 9-12 months of dating is the perfect amount of time to get to know each other extremely well, build trust, and establish boundaries. By this stage, you should be spending pretty much every night together anyway, so this is just taking it a step further, and you both should feel like you want to be with this person forever. If you aren't happy about moving in together, then you probably shouldn't do it.

One thing I didn't mention earlier was that you only progress onto the next stage on the relationship timeline if you are at a 10/10. You don't move in together if the relationship is an 8/10.

You cannot proceed further until the stage you are at is a 10/10. Some people believe having a baby together can save a relationship. Obviously, this is not true; it may give you two a deep bond, but after a few months the same problems come back up, and they seem even worse now because you have a baby together and you haven't dealt with the past. If the relationship is at a 10/10 and you both feel great about moving forward, then jump right in and have a beautiful life.

18-24 MONTHS

This is the time in the relationship to consider proposing or getting engaged to be married. This stage isn't as important on timing as the other stages are because you can always just take the ring off and everything is back to normal.

Guys, an important thing to remember with this is to never propose to a girl unless she is dropping hints to you or talking often about getting married. If she hasn't mentioned it at all and doesn't really seem that keen, then don't propose! Wait until she is dropping the hints, because then she's actually fully in love with you and ready to get married. Some women say "yes" to marriage even though they aren't ready; don't fall into this trap. Wait to see the signs.

Some men are such good leaders and so convincing that when they propose, the girl is thinking, "What the hell?" But she says "yes" anyway because he has a lot going for him, but she doesn't deeply love him yet. I've heard stories of women not falling in love with the guy until they have been married for like five years! Can you imagine that poor guy, going that entire time not realising that his wife didn't really want to get married?

So for that reason, wait for the hints. In a way, she should be asking you. Her hints will be extremely strong and loud; you won't miss them.

24-48 MONTHS

Marriage and Babies! After you are engaged and you have been together a few years, you know each other extremely well; this should be the stage where you start planning your wedding and babies if you are inclined that way. And anything that hap- pens after this is your choice. The timeline has finished. Please remember not to proceed to the next step on the relationship timeline unless you are at a 10/10 in your current phase. Jump- ing into the next step won't make your relationship better; it will just put more pressure on you as a couple. Guys, marriage and babies is a really great thing, but it is also a very feminine thing, so let your wife plan it all. You can help a bit, but it's mainly her thing, so don't be afraid to step back a little and lead from the back.

This chapter and concept is relatively short and easy to understand; however, remember you are the architect of your own life, and everything in this book is just a guide, so please modify any information you read to your specific circumstances or get in contact with me so I can help with your specific situation.

PART VI

Expanding on the Five Pillars

Hobbies

Most people when they first meet someone are flooded with positive emotions, and they start to fall in love. That feeling is lovely, and they think to themselves, "Well, I'm in love with this person, and now I'm going to clear my schedule for the next three months because all I want to do is spend time with this person."

Obviously not the best idea, but we all have done it in the past; that is why the relationship timeline is so important. Go back and reread the chapter on the relationship timeline if you need to. This chapter is about what hobbies you like to do, both by yourself and with your partner. Hobbies are a super import- ant part of life that most people forget about. They feel they are a waste of time, but on the contrary, they are extremely important for developing both our social skills and the feeling of community.

What I want you to do now is write down a list of ten hobbies/ activities you would like to try to do in the next six months.

For example, my ten are:

- Bodybuilding
- Karate
- Judo
- Tango
- Jet skiing
- Go-kart racing
- Gardening
- Swimming
- Writing children's books
- Toastmasters

I have done these things before, but I want to do them again and more often in the future. Doing lots of different hobbies makes for well-rounded rich human beings. I think we all know someone who is so boring; they just go to work, then come home, and that's all they do—they have no hobbies, no goals, no nothin'! Not a lot of fun to hang out with.

So you may be asking yourself, "Yes, hobbies are great, but why write about them in a relationship book?" Because so many people get into a relationship and forget about their hobbies. They lose themselves to the relationship, and after they change completely, then the person their partner fell in love with is gone. I've seen this countless times, and I've even succumbed to it in the past myself. So write down your top ten; you can change it over the years, but if you are anything like me, many of them stay the same. For example, I've loved bodybuilding and martial arts since I was a little kid and still do.

When should you do these hobbies? All the time. Do at least two to three different hobbies every week. Some hobbies you can do by yourself, others with your partner. For example, I do martial arts by myself, but I do tango, jet skiing, and gardening with my partner. I specifically pick hobbies my partner won't want to do, and vice versa. Encourage your partner to do hobbies you don't want to do. It is important to spend time with your partner, but it is also very important to spend time apart from your partner.

There isn't a person alive who you could spend 24/7 with and not get on each other's nerves. It's perfectly natural; that's why it's good to spend time with other people. Enjoy your hobbies, be social, and be part of the community.

What we do outside of work can often influence our success at work. Being in public service is extremely rewarding in many ways, but I do not have to tell you that it comes with its stresses too. Maintaining a healthy level of stress has many positive benefits, but there is a thin line between healthy and negative stress, which we all cross from time to time.

The way I have always handled excess stress is through my hobby. There are many health benefits to having a hobby, and it is also good for making friends, building confidence, and cultivating other skills that you may not get to work on as much at work. Let's take a look at why having a hobby is important:

5 REASONS EVERYONE SHOULD HAVE A HOBBY
1. CREATIVITY

Most hobbies require creativity, and developing creativity through a hobby can transfer directly into creativity at work. There are not many ways on the job to develop creativity, and this skill is extremely important in today's business world. When

I hire an employee, in job interviews I always ask people what they do for fun because it provides great insight into their personality, creativity, and passion. Gardening, baking, and all my hobbies really allow me to be creative in some way or another, especially in writing children's novels.

2. CONFIDENCE

Hobbies build confidence because being good at something and learning something new is very rewarding. Job roles and responsibilities change so frequently that we are often faced with learning new things. The confidence you gain from challenging yourself in your hobby can help prepare you for learning new things at work. My martial arts hobbies have given me tremendous confidence over the years, especially in violent situations in which I have found myself. A high confidence level is so important in life, leadership, and relationships.

1. REDUCE NEGATIVE STRESS

Getting caught up in something you enjoy doing is great for relieving stress because it refocuses your mind on something you enjoy. Hobbies that require some level of physical activity also create chemical changes in our body that help reduce stress, but even if your hobby does not require physical activity, you can still benefit. Getting a break from stress at work and doing something you enjoy can rejuvenate the mind and help better prepare you to handle challenges in the future.

1. SOCIALISE

The internet provides endless ways to connect with people that enjoy doing the same things you do. This is a great opportunity to meet new people, discuss your hobby, and get more involved with bigger groups. Many of my best friends are people I have met through my hobbies, and it is an easy way to make new friends when you travel or move to a new area. It is also a great way to make friends at work and in similar jobs at different organisations. I met one of my best friends at CrossFit. I don't do CrossFit anymore, but it was a great place to meet like- minded people and form great lifelong friendships.

5. PERSONAL DEVELOPMENT

I talked about creativity and confidence already, but personal development does not stop there. I learned many skills, such as video/photo editing, writing, photography, web design, etc... that were a complete byproduct of my hobby. This will happen to you too. You may end up running a local club, maintaining a website, creating flyers, helping with fundraisers, etc. These all translate into real skills you can use on the job. When I first started coaching people, my personal coach at the time rec- ommended I try Toastmasters, and I instantly fell in love with it. I originally went in to become a better public speaker, and even though I'm quite the confident speaker now, I still go to Toastmasters because it is enjoyable. The skills it teaches you are so vast, and billionaire Warren Buffet said public speaking is a skill everyone should learn.

TIPS ON SELECTING A HOBBY

If you do not already have a hobby or if you are looking at trying something new, there are a couple things to keep in mind. When you select a hobby, you want to consider the following:

CHALLENGING

Find something that is progressively more challenging but does not have such a huge learning curve that it will be years before you see any progress. Don't pick bodybuilding, because it is so hard and takes years to see anything decent.

FOCUS ON STRENGTHS

It is a good idea to focus on something that you have some natural ability at. If you are scared of heights, you would not try rock climbing, and if you don't like being outside, you probably would not take up mountain biking. Take into account your fitness level, finances, education, and passion when choosing a hobby.

STRESS

Take into consideration the level of stress of the hobby. One of my hobbies is playing Texas Hold'em, which has great qualities, but it is a very high-stress game. I have to balance that hobby with another one that has a lower level of stress. Getting past the beginner stage of a hobby can be stressful, but it does not take as long as you might think.

So, in conclusion, don't lose yourself in a relationship and forget who you are. Your partner fell in love with who you are, and if you change they might not like who you are anymore and, more importantly, you won't like who you are anymore either. You become a slave to the relationship, and your life starts to lose some of its beauty. It's time to start asking yourself the big questions in life, such as "Who am I?" and "What do I want?" You can achieve everything you want in life—and more. You

just need to get out of your own way and stop being a coward.
Give it 110 percent!

Children and Relationships

Do you have kids? Does your new partner have kids? This can be troublesome and lead to some issues within your relationship.

I have kids and my new partner doesn't. Many of my clients have children and stepchildren. This is very common, and it needs to be handled in the right way.

One of my clients, John, got into a relationship with a woman with three kids, and at times he found the kids to be quite naughty, and it seemed like they generally misbehaved a lot. Was it his place to say something? This is what we need to be careful of, guys: single mothers are very used to being mascu- line. They are used to being the dad and the mum at home. Now suddenly you're here and want to take over. This can disturb the natural order of things.

Guys, it needs to be done slowly. If you are a new man in the child's life, you will naturally become his father figure, but it will take time. Trust needs to be built with the child and the child's mother. Once this trust is established, then you will be able to be yourself and raise the child and have input. If you walk in on the first day of meeting the kids and start slapping them for being naughty, then the relationship will most likely end pretty fast. Take it slowly, treat them like friends at first, and lead by example.

Leading by example is a great way to build trust and to raise kids without them realising it. Make bonding activities that you all can do as a big family to build the relationship faster, and work hard on creating those opportunities. Men, still be the leader and create those opportunities. Don't sit back and let your girlfriend lead just because they aren't your kids.

Respect is extremely important. Even though at first you are going to come across to the child like you are their friend, you still never ever let anyone disrespect you. Have your boundaries that no one crosses, no matter what, regardless of their age or gender. If a five-year-old child who isn't yours is hitting you, then tell them to stop. You may feel mean doing this, but if you don't say anything you are disrespecting yourself and the child assumes you are weak. You really want to come across as strong and friendly.

A few of my clients have a child each, and then have gotten into a relationship together. They often find themselves saying things like "your child" and "my child." This is division, and it isn't good for a team or family. You need to act like they are both your children and say things like "the kids" or "our kids." As a leader, you need to make everyone feel included and emo- tionally safe. Emotional safety is the key to good leadership in a business or in a family. If you have a stepchild and you treat them with a kind of indifference like you would treat a stray dog, then the child will feel this level of neglect and they won't become the person they could've been with the right amount of love and attention.

When is the right time for your partner to meet your kids? If you remember back to the relationship timeline chapter, then you will remember that you don't go exclusive with someone until you have been dating for two to three months, and it takes two to three months to build trust and really get to know someone. Until you are in an exclusive relationship with someone and you have known them for at least three months, then don't introduce your kids to them. It is important that you are both in love with each other and the relationship is going well before the kids meet them.

If you are going out with someone who has kids and you eventually meet them, take some time. It will take a few months to get to know the children well, and over time you will fall in love with them, too, and consider them one of your own, and the children will feel emotionally safe around you and like they are part of your family.

One thing that I often see and have experienced myself is negative criticisms of the other parent. The other parent doesn't need to be your enemy just because they were in a relationship with your partner in the past. I'm not saying you need to be friends, either, but being nasty isn't helpful to anyone, and the kids will see that as well.

If your partner says something negative about their ex, just be quiet and try to remain neutral while still supporting your partner. Don't fan the flames of hatred. In these circumstances, you need to remember your common goal: you all want what is best for the children; you want them to grow up happy and strong. Unfortunately, everyone has a different opinion on how this should be done.

Firstly, there is no wrong answer as long as you all have the same goal. Everyone has a different parenting style and that's actually a good thing; it makes the child well-rounded and a good member of society. The term co-parenting is such bullshit. You don't need to be on the same page as your ex on raising the kids as long as you both have the same goal and you both want what's best for them. So many people argue about the littlest things with the ex-partners, and it's all rubbish. Disagreements don't matter; it's a good thing you have different methods of parenting.

One of the couples I coach, Josh and Brittany, have two small children, and they often disagree on the best way to raise them or discipline them. The first mistake they were making was that the mother was doing all the disciplining. This is a bad thing, girls. Being a disciplinarian is a masculine role and should be mainly done by the dad. I understand if you are a single mother and you have to try to do both, but if you are in a relationship, try to get your husband to do it. You need to step back and be mothering.

That's where all these terms came from: the mother should be mothering, feminine and kind, giving lots of hugs and kisses and all that sort of stuff, with no criticisms or bitchiness. The dad, on the other hand, is responsible for turning the child into a respectful member of society with good morals who knows the difference between right and wrong. He can also give hugs and kisses but not as much as the mother. He needs to be strong, lead his family to success, raise the kids, and teach them how to be strong, inside and out.

Mums getting in the way of training and discipline is a very common and natural thing. It's feminine to be mothering and want to protect your children, but this makes it very hard for the dad to do anything "dangerous or scary." I've been training my two sons in karate since they could walk, and I'll continue to do martial arts training with any kids I have in the future as well. I personally believe martial arts are really important and that it's very good to know how to defend yourself and others. When I train my sons, other people are allowed to watch, but I make them promise to be quiet or only say positive things. Anything negative will hurt the training process.

If I tell a young boy to do fifty push-ups, for example, and some-body tries to overrule me and say "No, no, fifty is too many, just do twenty," then that will negatively impact their growth. Yes, it is hard doing fifty push-ups for some people, unless you are used to it. It takes pain to grow in anything we do. Whether it's in the gym, martial arts, or business, if you want to become really good at something and you are willing to train at it, then you need to put your mind or body or both under pressure, because without pressure or pain, then you will not grow or improve.

Many cultures, like that of the Spartans, would train their boys away from their mothers because the mothers would hinder the training. There are some things in parenting that are difficult to do or watch, and disciplining is one of those things. If the child has been really bad and they need to be disciplined, it may be hard to witness, but remember if it is not done, then the child could turn into a spoiled, entitled brat. If you are the mum, and the dad is doing some disciplining, it is best if you remove yourself from the situation and go into the other room. It is the same with training. If the training is too hard to watch, then go into the other room. You need pressure to create diamonds. I know that may be hard to hear, and you may be triggered by this, but really ask yourself, "What sort of person do I want my child to grow up into? Do I want them to be a brat or a loser? Or do I want them to be strong and well-rounded?"

With parenting, try to stay within your natural energy. If you are female, stay feminine with the kids; if you are male, stay masculine. Almost every time a couple comes to me, the female is being super masculine with the kids and the male is being super feminine, and they wonder why they are having troubles. You may want a beautiful PC world where everything is equal and fair and nice, but that isn't reality. Real life and human beings are not like that! No matter how badly you want it, it won't happen! And to be honest, you may think you want it, but in reality you don't really because every single woman whom I have helped become more feminine has said she feels way better and it's so much easier, and the same is true for every man whom I help become more masculine. It is the natural order of things, and it works extremely well. You can't fight nature.

There have been some issues throughout history with domestic violence and men taking disciplining too far. This personally sickens me! That's why I live strictly to my sheepdog method, and that is the same method that everyone lives by in my house. The sheepdog method is this: There are three sorts of people in the world: sheep, sheepdogs, and wolves.

Sheep are people who can't defend themselves (think children or people of that nature). Then we have wolves, predators who take joy in hurting the sheep or hurting people who can't defend themselves (think bullying). Then we have sheepdogs, who protect the sheep and fight the wolves. We protect the weak from evil and preserve justice.

Everybody in my house is a sheepdog, and wolf-like behaviour will result in severe punishment and will never be accepted. Sheep behaviour is also not accepted, and victim-type mentality isn't welcome in my house, because we are strong, and we are sheepdogs. If you have children, then drill this into their heads from an early age, and it will pay off well; it's a super simple analogy that I live by strictly and that even a five-year-old could understand. If you don't have kids, then adopt this method for yourself anyway; it will improve your life and make the world a better place. I personally believe that even though this method is so simple, it could really change the world. Many people try to overcomplicate things and make this as complicated as possible when they don't need to. Albert Einstein said, "Make everything as simple as possible, but not simpler." It's a powerful sentence. Remember it.

Parenting is hard, but as long as your heart is in the right place, you will do okay. If you love your kids and you want them to turn out well, then listen to your gut—it knows what's right and wrong. It's our brain that messes everything up.

Long-Term Success

You have read every part of this book thoroughly, maybe even did the online course, but now, months later, you're thinking to yourself, "Damn, everything has gone back to the way it was! Our relationship is terrible again! What should I do?"

It's the same as exercise. You may get on a health kick and start eating really healthy and going to the gym a lot and you start looking really good, but then you think, "Well, I look great. I can relax a bit," and your body starts gaining fat again. Remember, there are no plateaus in life. You are either going up or down. Your relationship is getting better or worse. Your body, your business, everything is either going up or down. You decide which way it goes.

To ensure never-ending success in your life you must be fighting for growth, and fighting for improvement, because life really is a fight; there is no magic pill for success, and if you want a great body, great relationships, great finances, a great business, there is no shortcut. It's just hard work consistently over long periods of time. It's a long, hard road to success, so try not to focus so much on the destination. Try to enjoy the journey.

Ego is often one of the things that holds us back and hinders us from achieving a 10/10 relationship. Remember, you go into a relationship to give. If you are too focused on what you are getting out of the relationship, then it will never be a 10/10. If both people in the relationship are more focused on their partner rather than themselves, the relationship will be great. I know this may seem confusing because sometimes I say you need to put yourself first. The truth is you need to look after yourself first in a positive way so you can perform at your best in your relationship.

Another thing to remember is when you read a book, you only retain about 10 percent of the information, and even that small percentage dwindles over time. Because of this fact, you need to read this book at least fifteen times if you want to become a master at relationships. Then re-read it every six months after that. I've read some of my favourite books over fifty times because there is so much valuable information in them, and that is the reason for some of my success today.

Goals are so important in life and achievement. I honestly can't believe how few people have goals, and they seem to be just wandering through life aimlessly. You must have goals if you are going to achieve anything spectacular. I've always had rather ostentatious goals. Even from a very early age, I was very fixated on money, and by age ten, one of my goals was to be the richest person in the world. I understand not all people are wired the same and everybody is different. I understand I'm not normal in the way I think; however, that has given me quite an exciting, adventurous life and has allowed me to achieve so many goals, and will keep fueling me to achieve more and more. My goals are like oxygen; each breath is important but not as important as the next one. It's the same case for my goals; my next goal is always the most important.

If you don't have a clear plan on where you want to go, surely you will eventually find yourself somewhere you don't want to be. You need to have plans and goals for your relationship or love life. Many people may have a business plan or even some educational goals they want to achieve, but few have a relation- ship plan or goals. Relationships are a major part of human life. By just ignoring your love life, it won't ever turn into something good, so plan it out and put some work into it. Work on yourself and your relationships. The goals for your relationship don't need to be too complicated; they can be as simple as a small holiday here or there, a proposal on this date, a romantic gift on that date. This planning feels very weird and un-spontaneous. In saying that, people put way too much pressure on being sponta- neous, but it's not that important. You can plan something out a month in advance if you want to; then just keep it a secret, and your partner will think you're spontaneous, even though you planned that surprise gift months earlier.

Some people seem to struggle with being romantic, and they think it's extremely difficult. One of my clients bought his wife a teacup and gave it to her as a present. He didn't wrap the gift or do anything special, just bought it and gave it to her and said it was a present. I was shocked—that is so bad! Everyone, that is not a present! A romantic gift for your partner needs to be romantic and have some effort put into it. It must be wrapped, it needs to be a surprise, and you have to put some effort into the delivery.

Here are some quick tips to make your delivery more romantic: Head down to your local cheap shop and pick up one hundred tealight candles for one dollar. Make them into a love heart or something like that, and put a gift in the middle. Play some soft romantic music, maybe jazz in the background, and have some flowers around the gift as well. Then you need to work on the build-up. Make them close their eyes, slowly walk them into the room, and then make them wait, letting the suspense build and ultimately having a big reveal. You see? You can have a tonne of fun with delivery. A good delivery can make an average gift amazing, and a bad delivery can make a great gift terrible. Handing someone something unwrapped and saying "Oh, here you go, I bought you a gift" is the worst thing you can do. It shows you don't care at all, and you think you're too cool to put in any effort. Well, you may think you are too cool to put effort into gifts, but I bet you will put effort into your divorce lawyer. How cool will you feel then?

Remember there is no ego in love—it's open and free. If you have gotten to this stage in the book and you are still having trouble, it could mean a few things. It could be that you hav- en't taken action and done the things in the book, it could be you have taken some action and you just need to take more, it could be you just need more practice, or lastly and most sadly, it could mean the person you are in a relationship with isn't your ideal partner. You two may be so mismatched and have no similarities at all that even if you both become masters at relationships, you still won't get along. It's sad and unfortunate.

In some cases, two people just aren't meant to be together. Sometimes couples come to me and they have both cheated on each other over ten times, and there is obviously no trust there at all, yet they ask, "Can we be saved?" At that stage, after the amount of damage that has been done, it would be best if they just moved on and started again. If a house burns down, technically you could still live in it or put a tent up in the ashes, but it won't be the best home. Sometimes you need to bulldoze it away and start again. I don't see this that often, but if you are in a relationship and you believe way too much harm has been done to ever love or trust each other fully, then you need to just end the relationship and move on, because you can't make something great out of garbage. I hope you aren't in that type of situation and I can help you. Keep working hard at mastering relationships, and if the only thing you achieve in this life is having an amazing relationship, then I think it is a life well lived.

Long-term success and a successful life obviously mean concentrating on things outside your relationship as well—like business, health, finances, hobbies, and things of that nature. Realistically it's very hard to have a 10/10 relationship if your business is failing or you have extremely bad health. Say you have bad mental or physical health. It will come out in negative ways in your relationship, and negativity affects your overall score. So to have a 10/10 relationship, you have to work at all the other parts of your life as well. Become a well-rounded person and an inspiration to others.

Some people pester their partners to eat better foods or exer- cise more. Most people don't need pestering; in fact, that often results in the opposite of the desired effect happening. Lead by example. If you want your partner to eat better, then you eat better first. If you want your partner to exercise more, then you hit the gym every day and go for runs constantly. They will adopt better choices just because you are leading by example.

It just goes to show that communication is a funny thing, and often we try so hard to communicate and get our point across that they hate us for it and only negative things happen. If you communicate with your partner effectively, then they will feel motivated and inspired to listen and take your information on board, but if you communicate poorly, then your partner will feel criticised and belittled and negative, and nothing will change; instead, it will most likely just get worse.

I was talking to one female, Sarah, and she said she keeps dating guys and they keep cheating on her or turn out to be bad guys or whatever, and all guys are terrible, blah, blah, blah. Heaps of negative complaining and stuff like that. Now do you think that kind of talking will help her find her ideal partner or make it harder? Obviously, if you talk really negatively and have nothing but bad things to say about relationships and dating, then the universe will agree with you, and nothing positive will come into your life. So what sort of self-talk do you do?

Most people are self-sabotaging themselves somewhere. They will push their partner away or be mean to their partner and wonder what happened. They will think and say lots of nega- tive patterns and continue to live those negative patterns, truly believing the world is a bad place. Some people self-sabotage themselves when it comes to money or business. They may believe they don't deserve success or make truly stupid deci- sions. Many self-sabotage when it comes to love, and almost all the people who come to me know the right and wrong things to do in love and relationships, but they do the wrong thing and then think to themselves, "Damn, why did I do that?"

Often human beings are their own worst enemy, but I prefer to be my own best friend. Something to remember is that we have a very old brain that is always looking for problems to try to keep us safe. Think about what would happen if you did this in a relationship though. If you look hard enough in your relationship, you are bound to find lots of little problems, and as soon as you give those problems power, they turn into a cancer that slowly destroys the relationship, and it can all start from something so small like a text from the opposite sex or an ex-partner. This is why we need to constantly be working on ourselves, our confidence and self-esteem, and our overall health. If we have low confidence, then it will be very hard to achieve a 10/10 relationship because we will overreact to every- thing that has the potential to harm us.

Often people attract what they fear. Men often do this if they are super worried that their partner is going to cheat on them. They give that fear so much energy and power that they start to manifest it happening, and their own insecurities push their partner away into the arms of someone else, and they do end up cheating. I see it all the time, but it's not their fault. No one has taught them about relationships, so all they have to go off is their parents or movies, which are not the best way to learn. Instead of manifesting negativity, fear, or bad things to happen, manifest positivity, success, and love. Constantly say and think positive things about your partner and love life, and the good will just get brighter.

You can do this with almost every part of your life. You are the architect of your own life. Design it exactly how you want it to be. If someone, anyone, is hurting your chances of long-term success, then they have to go, even if that person is your part- ner. If you want a 10/10 relationship and your partner keeps doing and saying things that are taking you off the path to success, then you need to realise this person probably isn't your ideal partner; they are simply too much work, and it's time to move on.

Anything or anyone hindering your goals has got to go. Really, that is the key to long-term success: surrounding yourself with people who help you achieve your goals, not hinder them. The majority of people surround themselves with people who hinder their goals. They tell them their goals are stupid and a waste of time, and the really bad thing is the person usually listens to their "friends." Now, if you really think about it, would your friends say all these negative things to you or would they sup- port you? Would your ideal partner do things that would help your relationship get to a 10/10, or would they do things that would hurt it?

In conclusion, if you are still having trouble, reach out to me. Send me a message or an email or contact me any way you can, and I will try to help. My main goal in life is to help as many people as I can with relationships. If I can help you in any way, please let me know. You can achieve a 10/10 relationship. I wrote this book to help you achieve a 10/10 relationship, and if you use this book effectively, then you will succeed.

About the Author

Clearly you can see I am very passionate about relationships. I plan on writing many relationship books, as I truly believe it is the key to living a great life. I am married to my beautiful wife, Tori Maddock, who is an absolute angel, and our relationship is a 10/10 and always has been and constantly improves each year. I will be with her until I die. I am thoroughly enjoying building a family and wonderful life with her. With her sup- port, I have become very successful. To the men reading this, do you want to be really successful? Find the perfect woman to support your goals.

I grew up in a large family. I have seven brothers and sisters. My family is not close at all, and my parents' relationship isn't very good and never was. I've done lots of different things over the years. I was in the army for years, and it was amazing—thoroughly recommended for all men under the age of twenty-one. I was always passionate about relationships and studied them through the years. It truly is my passion, and I will coach people on relationships for the rest of my life.

While writing this book, I have been a relationship coach

for about Six years. I'm so passionate about this. I do it one hundred hours a week, and I never get tired because I am so enthusiastic about relationships. With all this hard work and the thousands I have coached so far, it feels like I've only just started. Much, much more to come, folks, so pay attention.

www.ingramcontent.com/pod-product-compliance
Lightning Source LLC
Chambersburg PA
CBHW051722260326
41914CB00031B/1695/J